Praise for Fearless Birthing

A step on from hypnobirthing

Best book I've read about birthing and this is my third baby. It's the one book I'd recommend.

Charlie, Amazon reviewer

Fearless Birthing is **a must read for all mums-to-be** who are looking to create a positive mindset for their birth. Alongside Alexia's work on her podcast and website, this book details a unique method of clearing fears in preparation for childbirth. It is **easy to read** and to follow along with the clearance method and also provides a lot of background info on the technique.

Alexia's work has helped me immensely in my birth preparation - truly a fantastic guide!

Gemma Croft, Expecting baby #1

Having been a long term fan of Alexia's *Fear Free Childbirth* podcast I was so excited to hear about her new book, and **it doesn't disappoint!** Alexia's style is chatty, informative and easy-to-read with the huge bonus being the tool she has developed that empowers women to reduce their fear levels in pregnancy and birth. **This is a great signpost for anyone who wants to take responsibility for her birth** experience and clear some head trash!

Sophie Brigstocke, Doula of the year 2017

This book is a fabulous tool. **Not only for expectant parents**, no matter how many previous births they've experienced, but **also for birth workers**. And I feel like this book is very versatile. As in, no matter what birthing technique - Hypnobirthing, Bradley method, Lamaze, etc - or if you've scheduled a cesarean birth.

I highly recommend this book for parents to have the most positive birth experience possible. As a doula, I feel this book has wonderful information on how to help my clients clear their fears surrounding births, and my own fears so I can support these women in the best way I can.

Skie Fortier, Doula

I was thrilled to find out that we were expecting, but also fearful of the pain and complications that would come with birth. The anxiety that I felt from the preconceived amount of pain that was to come in delivery was making me stress so much that I was having a difficult time enjoying pregnancy. I feel so fortunate to have found Alexia's Fear Free Childbirth Podcast and to have had the opportunity to read Fearless Birthing to help me understand my fears, where they were coming from, and how to clear them.

Reading the book was like sitting down to tea with a dear friend that is honest and understanding of your fears. This book changed my outlook on birth and made me realize that all of my fears were completely normal, and I just needed to learn how to clear them. Alexia is authentic in her writing and doesn't attempt to push beliefs onto you, rather she shows you options backed by research and stresses the importance of doing what is right for your birthing experience. There were so many gems in this book that really opened my eyes to how wonderful birth can be instead of fearing the countdown.

Nikki Coleman, Expecting baby #1

Fearless Birthing demonstrates how to harness the power of your mind to improve your pregnancy and birth. Alexia guides you on ridding your mind of the conscious and sub-conscious negative patterns ['head trash'] not serving you and appreciates that big or small, clearing them will reduce your overall stress levels. Alexia's ultimate goal for you is a positive birthing experience that you will fondly remember always, and she shows you multiple ways to achieve this.

Kristen Soloway, Planning her pregnancy

Upon reading the book's first words I could hear Alexia's voice speaking. Which, when I've listened to her podcasts is always full of energy, emotion and general good vibes, even when serious topics are discussed. As she shares her own journey of pregnancy and birth it reminds the reader that she are not just writing from a therapist point of view. I found most of her statistical information to be spoken in a way that most readers will be able to follow and identify easily with especially if they've experienced pregnancy and birth previously.

As a birth professional I found her step-by-step instructions quite helpful in organizing my thoughts for how best to have helpful and encouraging discussions with clients who may be struggling with fears or concerns. Though one doesn't need to be a provider or therapist of course to do this.

She has written this for women to do their own head trash clearance and I think this book will help many women do just that. In *Fearless Birthing* she has laid out a map with easy to follow instructions and advisement when to seek outside professional help. While using both anecdotal and researched evidence. She's written in a way that is engaging and real for the reader.

I will definitely be putting this book on my recommendation list and especially for women who are struggling with fear or anxiety with their pregnancy and upcoming birth."

I really enjoyed reading this book. I especially loved learning about the fear-clearance technique. I am a mental health professional and really enjoyed exploring alternatives to traditional therapies in order to overcome fears. I've done one fear clearing since reading the book and was amazed at the response I got. I can't wait to be able to do more clearings in order to prepare for my upcoming birth.

Jackie LeBreck, Expecting baby #2

Fearless Birthing has been so helpful in learning to confront and clear my fears. Not only that, but it really helped me to pinpoint exactly what those fears were to begin with which I previously couldn't even figure out. Alexia provides a great deal of helpful information about pregnancy, labor, and childbirth and I loved reading about her personal experiences.

I found this book very empowering as I truly believe using the methods in it will help me to make the right decisions about my labor and birth and it has already helped me feel like my body is not only capable of this, but made to do this. I plan to continue to refer to this book and to work on fear clearing as I finish out these last few weeks of pregnancy. I am now actually looking forward to going into labor with confidence and much less "head trash".

Amanda Zagunis, Expecting baby #3

FEARLESS BIRTHING

Clear Your Fears For a Positive Birth

ALEXIA LEACHMAN

mankai media

Published by Mankai Media, UK.

For permission requests or bulk orders contact the publisher by writing to hello@mankaimedia.com

Visit the author's websites at fearless-birthing.com and www.alexialeachman.com

First edition.

ISBN 978-1-9998915-1-0

Disclaimer: This book is designed to provide helpful information on pregnancy and birth. It doesn't constitute medical advice or an alternative to appropriate medical care, nor is in any way a guarantee or promise of expected, imagined or actual outcome of labour or birth. It is not the substitute for the advice or the presence during birth any part of pregnancy or labour of a qualified medical practitioner, midwife or obstetrician.

The Fearless Birthing method and this book describing its techniques are not intended to represent a medically and anatomically precise overview of pregnancy and birthing, nor are they designed to represent medical advice or a prescription for a medical procedure. The content of this book is not intended to replace the advice of a medical doctor. It is advisable for any pregnant woman to seek the advice of a medical doctor or healthcare provider before undertaking any pregnancy or labour-related program.

Persons following any course of action recommended in this book or in the Fearless Birthing method do so of their own free will. The author, the publisher assume no responsibility for any possible complications related to either the pregnancy or the labour of the participant. Every effort has been made to ensure all information in this book is correct. Any unintended error will be corrected in the next edition.

Credits: Book cover design by Andy Briscoe and editing by Sasha Tropp.

To Lila & Sofia

My inspiration and my greatest teachers.
You both taught me so much before you even drew a breath.

Life consists not in holding good cards but in playing those you hold well.

Josh Billings

Contents

Chapter Eleven

Chapter Twelve

Chapter Thirteen

Chapter Fourteen

Chapter Fifteen

Preface

The first time I found out that I was pregnant it hit me like a kick in the stomach.

The best way to describe my reaction was utter shock, mixed in with a massive dose of fear and terror. *Shock* because it wasn't consciously planned; *fear* and *terror* because the whole idea of being pregnant was utterly terrifying. During those first few weeks of my pregnancy I was an emotional mess. My doctor and midwife couldn't figure out my due date because I had no idea when my last period was; I was travelling around South East Asia at the time and I think I was in Vietnam. So I spent those first few weeks in and out of hospitals getting dating scans pretty much every week.

It was our fourth visit when we got the news: we had lost the baby. Cue second kick in the stomach. I was crushed. Just as I was starting to get my head around being pregnant, it was all over. The little one barely made it past eight weeks, and now I had to deal with all the messiness that comes with a miscarriage. It was a pretty dark time full of confusion and turmoil. The loss was unbearable, and yet a tiny part of me was relieved. Relieved because *then I didn't need to go through with the birth*. That bit scared me - surely not a healthy maternal response. This was head trash on a monumental scale.

I knew I had head trash - rampant negative thoughts, feelings, and emotions - but this was a sign. And a big one at that. A sign that I needed to probe and poke into my headspace and figure out what the hell was going on: *what was it that made me feel relieved at experiencing a miscarriage?*

As a mindset coach, this bothered me. If I were one of my clients, I'd be encouraging myself to get to the bottom of this. I was already trained in a number of mindset shifting techniques, but this was eluding me. Then it seems that my prayers were answered. One day I was having lunch with my good friend Pam, and she told me about this brand new therapeutic technique: "Alexia, I know you'll just love it . . . the first training course is in a couple of months - why don't you do it?" If I believed in God, that moment would have had him booming down at me in all his white beardiness: "GO! Go take the course!" The pull I felt was incredible, like it was my destiny! So I did.

This new therapy was called *Reflective Repatterning*, and it was mind-blowing, let me tell you. And life changing. Over the years I had tried all sorts of interventions in an attempt to sort out my head, but Reflective Repatterning finally made serious headway. And it was fast! I hate faffing about, so this was good for me. I think I got addicted to it; clearing my head trash, that is. When you start getting results that feel so transformational, you don't want to stop. Or at least that how things went for me. In the months that followed my miscarriage, I spent a lot of my time using it to address the things I was struggling with in my head. It was the beginning of a whole new phase of my life, wherein I was stripping back all the unhelpful conditioning that I'd absorbed through life and was rediscovering and reconnecting to who I was. Like I said: *transformational.*

Fast-forward a year and I found out I was pregnant again. Thankfully, this time I wasn't shocked. A lot had changed in that year. For starters, my partner and I had The Kids Conversation; you know the one, where you talk about having kids or not? Our miscarriage made us realise that we both wanted kids. It also made us realise that we were not ready by any stretch of the imagination. We were on the verge of moving to London, but when I got pregnant we parked that idea and decided to stay where we were and buy a family home. The sale went through just before we found out about the miscarriage. We bought the house at an auction, so suddenly we had a huge refurbishing project on our hands. The rest of the time I was focussed on sorting my head out. If I was going to be a mother, I needed to shed my extreme levels of stress and anxiety.

Over the years I'd read how maternal stress affects the unborn baby. As someone who grew up with the holy trinity of afflictions (eczema, hay fever, asthma) and allergies (dogs, cats, dust, feathers, horses, etc.), over the years I'd come across quite a bit of research that suggests that conditions like this are as a result of the mother being stressed while carrying her baby. I knew for sure that my mum was super stressed when she was carrying me. I didn't want to take any chances with my own child. Having eczema, asthma, and allergies sucks; it affected my self-esteem and my confidence. At school I was picked on and bullied because of it, I couldn't do certain sports, we couldn't have pets. Well, you get the picture! Thankfully I was now trained in a therapy that I knew could help me with all this. Banishing my stress was important if I wanted to do the best thing for my baby. So you could say that I was 110% keen to do everything I could to prevent my own child afflicted by the health challenges that I had. And for me, this meant having a stress-free pregnancy. In my current stressed state, this seemed like a mother of a mountain to climb, but it was important enough for me to give it a go.

I have to say, I made brilliant progress and my overall levels of stress and anxiety reduced massively that year. I'd taken a proper hard look at myself and made some changes. I did a bit of digging in the recesses of my mind and emotional landscape, and I'd found a load of stuff that wasn't entirely pretty. It wasn't easy. So yeah, I faced some demons and duly slain them too. But it was working: I was sleeping better, my confidence had improved, and I was coping with life's curveballs much better. I was more emotionally resilient. I guess this helps to explain why when I found out I was pregnant for the second time, that I was able to experience joy instead of shock. But I still had a ton of stress and anxiety in the *pregnancy-childbirth-motherhood* department, because I still felt like I was being stalked by this bloodcurdling fear.

I tried to figure out what was going on. *What was the problem? Why was I so scared?* I slowly came to realise that it was pregnancy that was freaking me out. *A thing growing inside me?* Yikes! But even more terrifying was the birth. I was terrified at the thought of childbirth. But was it that? *Was it the actual birth? Was it because it represented the beginning of motherhood? Was I reliving some deeply buried prior trauma?* I had no idea. All I was sure of was the hollow, sick feeling I felt inside, and the weird compulsion to cry every time any aspect of birth was mentioned. Whenever I thought about birth, I'd tense up and cross my legs as I tried to block out that awful video I had been shown in school, of a woman screaming in agony as she gave birth. Not only that, but every time I read about a birth I would well up and cry, not really knowing why. You know those stories that crop up every now and then, about women giving birth in cars or at airports because things happened so quickly? Well, if I came across one of those stories in a newspaper while on the train I'd just start crying. Weird right? There was clearly something not right in my emotional world when it came to birth.

This just reinforced my sense that I had *serious issues*! Remember, I was the one who was relieved at having a miscarriage. But then this other part of me figured it was pretty normal. Birth was a horrible, painful experience, right? We all know that! Didn't most women fear giving birth? Whether it was normal or not, I had to sort this out, because if I didn't, I was going to be in a right mess.

As luck would have it, I was due for another Reflective Repatterning training course. It was time for the advanced course, which happened to coincide with the start of my second trimester. The great thing about therapy training is that you get to air your dirty laundry in a safe place. So the time came for us to share our fears and stresses so that we could practice clearing them. As a terrified, fearful thing, this was great news; I had carte blanche to tell anyone who'd listen all about my childbirth fears and terrors. Up until that point I thought I just had to put up with them, and so I had pretty much decided to have a highly medicalised birth with all the drugs and injections I could get my hands on, anything that would help me cope with the PAIN! I was even seriously contemplating a C-section, just to avoid it all together.

A chance conversation during a coffee break changed everything for me. Julie, the wife of the course organiser, told me that there was no need to be worried about pain, because it was possible to have a natural, pain-free birth. *Natural* as in no drugs. I laughed as you do when you're not quite sure if someone is pulling your leg. "How on earth did you do that?!" I asked.

"Hypnobirthing," she replied.

Well, that was it. Once I knew there was another way, I wanted to find out all about it and so began my own educational journey about birth. The big question in my mind was this: *how is it possible NOT to experience pain during labour?* I also wanted to find out all about this *hypnobirthing* thing. So I dove head-first into my hypnobirthing phase; I diligently read the books and listened to all MP3 sessions I could get my hands on. All of it. But you know what? I still had THE FEAR! Hypnobirthing helped me in lots of ways because it opened up a whole new world of birth education that I seriously needed. The most important thing I learned was this: when it comes to childbirth, fear increases your chances of experiencing pain. But my deepest, darkest fears around childbirth were still there; my stuff was *deep*. It was so deep-rooted that even *I* didn't know what it was. I came to the conclusion that I probably needed to have some private sessions to sort this out because it was eluding me.

But then it hit me. I knew that my deeply felt fears needed some hardcore clearance action, and that's just what Reflective Repatterning is good at - clearing out negative thoughts, feelings, and emotions. So I decided to apply Reflective Repatterning not only to my goal of having a *stress-free pregnancy*, but also to my new goal of a *fear-free birth*. My mother of a mountain just became colossal! But I knew it must be possible, so I got to it.

During the rest of my pregnancy, I made some tweaks to Reflective Repatterning so that I could use it on myself quickly and easily. I wanted to prepare my mind and my body for a fear-free birth, which if

I'd understood the theory correctly, meant that gave me a chance of avoiding pain. It was worth a try, right? I was basically using myself as a guinea pig because no one had prepared for birth just using Reflective Repatterning before (especially my tweaked version of it!); it was such a new therapy, I was the first pregnant Reflective Repatterning graduate to try it out. It wasn't easy, because normally when you have therapy, you go and see someone and have a two-way conversation *with another person*. But only a handful of us were trained in this worldwide, and I had a mountain of fears and stresses to get through. I had to find a way to self-treat. So I tinkered with the technique and made some changes. I also created recordings for each of my fears for me to listen to and clear in turn so that I could pretend I was with a therapist. It took time and effort, let me tell you! But guess what? I did it! By month eight I decided to change my birth plan to home birth and I felt like I could totally do it. I had my first daughter at home and it was amazing. And, hand on my heart, it was *pain-free*. It was intense and hard work, for sure. But no pain. IT WORKED!

Of course, once I'd had my daughter, I wanted to share what I'd learned from the top of my metaphorical mountain, but I didn't. *What if it was a fluke? Maybe it had nothing to do with all the work I did. Perhaps I was just lucky.* All my self-doubt head trash started piling in. So I kept it to myself, only sharing it with people I knew (who got some great results). I pretty much left all my work to gather digital dust on my hard drive.

When I found out I was pregnant again a few years later, I knew it was my chance to see if my stuff really did work. I *needed* it to! I still hated the thought of pain, and I wasn't sure I could face the kind of birthing experience I'd read in the horror section. *Can I repeat my first childbirth experience? What if I have complications? What about my fears? Will they come back? And what about my stress levels during my pregnancy? What will they be like this time? What if I can't repeat my birthing experience?* Even though I knew a pain-free birth was possible, every pregnancy and birth is different, so there were no guarantees. As it happened, I had a whole different heap of stresses to deal with this time, and a load of new fears, which meant tons more clearance work.

Thankfully, as well as now being a lot more experienced at clearing head trash, I'd also learned a load of new therapies, methods and approaches for mind and body, so I had some new stuff to add to the mix. So what happened? Well, I did it again. Except this time it was even better. I didn't think I could beat my first birth, but I did. The birth of my second daughter was pretty magical in lots of ways. But it wasn't only pain-free, it was euphoric too, which I was NOT expecting!

At the time, I didn't realise that my journey and what I had achieved was a big deal. I thought I had just managed to side-step another of life's curveballs that affected fearful weirdos like me, of which there couldn't be many. It only became apparent to me once I started getting bombarded with emails from pregnant women - who I didn't know! - friends of friends and who'd heard about what I'd done and the births I'd had as a result. They wanted to know how I'd gone from fearful to fearless; what I did and how I did it. It got to the point that I reached the only possible conclusion: writing a book would be quicker than responding to all those emails.

I started writing when my baby was five weeks old and completed my first draft in about three months. Then I thought, "Hey, wouldn't it be a great idea if I shared some of this stuff via a podcast?" I figured it would be quicker than getting a book published. And, more importantly, I still had some pregnant friends waiting for my promise of a reply to their email! So that's why I decided to launch the *Fear Free Childbirth* podcast. It was just meant to be this little maternity-leave side project before going back to my Head Trash business.

The *Fear Free Childbirth* podcast quickly took on a life of its own. My other podcast, *The Head Trash Show*, was a pretty successful one. It was nominated for an international podcasting award in Las Vegas, and was regularly at the top of the self-help charts on iTunes. But *Fear Free Childbirth* was something else. The download numbers quickly eclipsed *The Head Trash Show*, and it was also nominated for a podcasting award here in the UK. I quickly started getting loads of emails from all over the world from my listeners, telling me how much the podcast had changed their lives. I was a bit slow to pick up on the signs, but I got the message eventually: I needed to take this seriously.

So I parked the book and threw myself into the podcast and seeking out brilliant guests for the show. I also revisited everything I'd created during my first pregnancy that had helped me to get over the bulk of my childbirth fears, to see how I could share it in a way that allowed other women to follow the exact same steps I did. The result was *Fearless Birthing Academy*, an online programme that teaches women how to prepare for their fearless birth. It wasn't long before I was being approached by birthing professionals who wanted to learn my fear-clearance method so that they could use it with their clients. This prompted me to create a training course and I ran my first pilot programme for *Fearless Birthing Professionals.*

By the time I'd got back to the book, I realised how much more I'd learned about working with women with a fear of birth. My first draft was written by a mum sharing her journey, but by the time I came round to editing it, I had become a birth professional myself. Since writing the draft I've been sharing my fear-clearance method and I've had so many women tell me how much it's helped them, that I now know for sure that it works - I'm not some special snowflake! So I guess I've proved to myself that that my first childbirth wasn't a fluke and that my fear-clearance approach works.

I know only too well that there are a lot women out there who are desperate for a positive birthing experience, but who are so full of fear. Many of them have had difficult first births and want to do anything they can to shed their fear of it happening again. Others are first-time mums who have heard so many horror stories that they feel over-whelmed, with some even experiencing prenatal depression. Some are not even pregnant yet, but they want to be. But their fear holds them back. This book is for them.

Sure, it's taken me a while; as I write this my youngest daughter is now coming up to her third birthday, but I'm now ready to birth *this* baby!

So, ladies - here it is!

Alexia, October 2017

Who Is This Book For?

This book is for you, if...

You're pregnant or trying to get pregnant and:

- The thought of childbirth scares you
- You suffer from tokophobia, the extreme fear of childbirth and pregnancy
- You are open to idea that it *is* possible to experience a pleasurable or pain-free birth, and wonder how that might be achievable
- You're keen to learn more about childbirth and the options available to you
- You would like to do what you can to make your birthing experience as positive as possible
- You're in a healthy state of mind and body
- You've read about conscious parenting and would like to start preparing to be a conscious parent during your pregnancy journey
- You want to use your pregnancy journey as an opportunity

to clear out your negative emotional patterns in preparation for parenthood

You're a guy and your wife or girlfriend is pregnant, and you both want to experience a fearless birth.

You're a birth worker and you're looking for ways to better support the families you serve who might be fearful about birth.

You're a sceptic who's curious as to how on earth it might be possible to have a pain-free birth and you're open to finding out.

This book is NOT for you if...

- You're looking for a quick fix
- You're not willing to put in the time and effort
- You're not prepared to take a look in the mirror

How to Use This Book

You can read this book in any way you choose, so if you feel drawn to particular sections, then go right ahead and dive in. However, if you'd like to take a deliberate and conscious journey to a fear-free birth, then I recommend you start by reading through the book in the order I've set out. Once you've done that, it's quite likely that you'll jump back to sections you need to revisit.

The fear-clearance journey is not a linear one; if I were to draw it, it would probably do a loop-the-loop across the page, with highs and lows, and parts where you find yourself feeling like you're going backwards before being thrust forwards. Much like a rollercoaster! But as with all journeys we embark on, it can be super useful to get a sense of the road ahead, so that you can relax and settle into it, which is why I encourage you, at least for the first time, to read the book in order.

This is designed to be a practical book - it's a how-to after all - so there are parts where you will be invited to do some work. At first, this "work" will involve thinking and self-reflection, but don't be fooled into assuming that this early stuff isn't important and can be skipped . . . especially if you are committed to the fearless birthing journey. This introspection is extremely important, and forms part of the very fabric of a conscious pregnancy. The more time and effort you spend on this self-reflection the better, because it will help you be more effective at clearance later. So, onto that: the clearance work. The central part of this book is about getting rid of your fears, so as the book goes on, I show you how to clear them. This requires a little bit more than self-reflection; it requires commitment and consistency if you are to achieve results. So please don't think that merely reading this book will clear your fears. I can show you the path, but you have to walk along it on your own steam.

Additional Resources

During the course of the book I share a bunch of tools and tips that can help you on your clearance journey. To help you with this I have created some resources which you can find in the online area that accompanies the book. I'm talking things like handy sheets to help you do the work I suggest. If you're anything like me, then having some nice printouts just makes it more likely for me to sit down and do the work. So if this does it for you, brilliant!

I'm also giving you a free Fearless Birthing Meditation, so that you can experience a broad level of fear clearance around pregnancy and birth before you dive down deeper to tackle your own individual fears. Hearing the fear-clearance method in action by listening to the meditation, should make it much easier to apply it to your own fears.

To gain access to your online area visit here to sign up www.fearlessbirthing.academy/book-resources

But that's not all: I also share some shortcuts with you, because let's be honest - who doesn't like a shortcut? I know how much work is required to clear the emotional decks in preparing for birth, and I know that not everyone has the time to do this. So I've created some shortcuts to help you on your journey. But *DISCLAIMER ALERT* they're not all free. It's up to you whether you're happy getting on with the work at hand, or whether you'd prefer to get there a little more quickly. It's as if you can decide to walk into town or pay for the bus: I'll tell you about the bus route, but you don't *have* to take it.

Finally, I think it's super important to talk about the other things you need to consider as part of your fearless birthing journey, things that will help when done alongside this book. Here are a few to consider:

1. STOP watching birthing reality shows! I'll name no names, but you know the type of shows I mean.
2. LIMIT the time and energy you spend with people who are negative about birth, whether they are sharing their birthing horror stories or telling you how tough you'll find it.
3. THINK CAREFULLY before sharing too much about your birthing plans; some people will be quick to judge and tear you down, especially the well-meaning friends and family who think they are only doing so to protect or prepare you.
4. FIND a supportive group of people who are open to the idea of a positive, fear-free birth. This might be hard in person, so look online. There are plenty of supportive Facebook groups, including mine ("Fear Free Childbirth").
5. SEEK OUT positive birth stories. My *Fear Free Childbirth* podcast is a great place to start if you want to hear women talking about their positive birthing experiences. There are also some fabulous websites and Facebook groups where women share countless positive birth stories.

What to Expect ...

... AND WHAT NOT TO EXPECT.

A positive pregnancy and childbirth experience takes time and effort

Removing the emotional and stress triggers in your life to enable you to enjoy a stress-free pregnancy will take more time and effort than simply reading this book. Just like with a marathon, you can read training plans all you like, but it's the hard slog of putting your trainers on and getting out there and running, consistently, that will get you over the finish line. The same goes for preparing for childbirth. Childbirth is a demanding experience both physically and emotionally - it's not called labour for nothing! If you want to be free of fear on the Big Day, then your body and mind will need to be prepared adequately. This book will show you how to handle the mental and emotional preparation, but only you can do the actual work.

This book is NOT a guarantee

While this book will show you the route, it does not guarantee that you will get there. Even if you do all the work, there are a ton of reasons why you might not be able to achieve your goal of stress-free pregnancy and fear-free childbirth. For starters:

- Your doctors consider you high risk given what they know about you and your lifestyle
- You suffer from medical conditions that are known to cause potential problems for pregnancy or childbirth
- Your health is not in an optimal state . . . for example, you may be overweight, have diabetes, or addicted to drink or drugs
- You suffer from mental health issues
- Your baby has other ideas

These examples don't mean that it's not possible for you; they simply mean that I can't make any promises. However, if you're in a reasonably healthy state of mind and body and your pregnancy is going well, then there is no reason why a fear-free pregnancy and birth shouldn't be possible for you.

This book promotes a holistic approach

We're an interconnected system, a body that's influenced by the mind, and a mind that's influenced by the body. Our conscious mind is affected by our subconscious, and our body is affected by both. So although this book won't teach you what to do with your *body* to prepare for childbirth, its advice is based on the belief and assumption that we are able to influence our body through the mind, and vice versa.

I am NOT a doctor, midwife, or doula

This book contains everything that I've learned as a result of my journey of my three pregnancies and two childbirths. I am a therapeutic coach and I do not claim to be qualified in medical or midwifery matters. Instead, my perspective is of a woman who started her pregnancy journey as someone who was utterly terrified of having kids and giving birth, and who went on to have two incredible births that were free of stress and fear. It's been an intense journey that involved a lot of time spent learning, reading, researching, and trying out countless ideas. During my pregnancies, the information I wanted and needed was very hard to find. I had to dig deep into Google and read a lot of scientific research papers to get the answers I needed to help me feel confident in my decisions (much of which is shared in the pages of this book). I have spent over eight years developing concepts, and have tested them on myself and willing friends and friends-of-friends. My efforts and work has been put to the test twice during both my births. What I'm sharing with you is a culmination of my own quest for answers and solutions to the challenges I was facing. My hope is that my journey and experience can help to inform yours.

This book is a HOW-TO guide

If you choose to, you can use this book as a guide to help you to clear your fears and stresses around pregnancy and childbirth. The first part of this book helps you to address fears that you might have as a result of not knowing much about the birthing process, so it's more informative in nature. If you still have fears after reading that, then the next part of the book is more practical and shows you how to clear individual fears and stresses. I also include lots of shortcuts.

This book is part of a much bigger whole

When I finished the first draft of this book I decided to start the *Fear Free Childbirth* podcast because I thought it would be a quicker way of sharing the key concepts of the book (publishing a book takes time!). The podcast is a mix of interviews with birth experts, mothers telling their positive birth stories and me sharing mindset tips and strategies for birth preparation. Today it's been downloaded over 330,000 times in over 180 countries and it's credited with helping women to completely shift their mindset when it come to birth preparation. The success of the podcast (and the mountains of emails I received from my listeners) encouraged me to develop more to support women in releasing their fears and preparing for a positive birth. Today these include;

Fear-clearance meditations are audio sessions that address specific fears. You receive one with this book, but there is a whole collection of them.

Fearless Birthing Academy is my online programme to accompany this book. It includes videos, audios and worksheets to help you to prepare for your positive birth. While some people are happy to crack on with following instructions in a book, some people need more and this is for them. There's also a Tokophobia version called the *Tokophobia Support Program*.

Fearless Mama Ship is my ultimate online resource of birth planning and preparation resources to help you to become a fearless mama. Preparing for a positive birth is so much more than simply getting rid of your fears. It's also about learning about birth and doing the necessary preparation and planning. But this kind of work doesn't stop the day your baby is born; birth is just the beginning!

Fearless Birthing Professional Training which is my training for doulas, midwives and therapists in the Fearless Birthing method so that they can use it with the women in their care.

I wrote this book to be used by pregnant women to clear their head trash around their pregnancy and birth. This book outlines the exact steps I took to achieve my fearless births. The thing is, I'm lazy. I'm also a huge fan of figuring out how to make things better, stronger, and faster, and this has led me to create some tools and shortcuts to help make the Fearless Birthing journey a little bit easier (just in case I had to do it again some day!). Many of these now form part of the various programmes that I've created. When I did this, there were no shortcuts, because no one had done what I was doing before; no one had applied this new therapeutic technique to pregnancy and birth. But now that I've figured it out, I've created some tools and shortcuts to make all this quicker and easier.

At certain points during the book I will mention things I've come up with that will save you time or offer you additional support if that's what you need. Feel free to ignore them. What I share in this book is exactly how I achieved my fearless birth. If shortcuts are your thing, then you'll probably appreciate me sharing them with you. If I have created products, tools, or resources to take some of that work off your hands, then I will mention them, because I know how long this stuff takes to do, and I want to help you to get results. I also know how busy people can be, especially if your sleep requirement has just shot up to ten hours a day, like mine did. Equally, if there are aspects in which I'm able to support you more closely in your journey, then I'll mention those too.

So, if you're the kind of person who will curse me for mentioning my products or services, then please let me ask for your forgiveness right now. My only intention is to help you.

Head Trash

As well as being the name of the business I had before baby number two,"Head Trash" is the term I use to describe *negative thoughts, feelings, and emotions* that prevent you from experiencing the life you want. As such, I use that term all the time. I'll try not to use it too much in these pages, as I realise that it won't mean as much to you as it does to me, but I will, if only because I'm pretty lazy and can't bear the thought of constantly typing out the words *negative thoughts, feelings, and emotions*. It would probably sound a bit repetitive too. So occasionally I'll use *head trash* instead written in small letters (Head Trash in caps refers to my work). And when I do, that's what I'm talking about: all that mental noise. The limiting beliefs that hold you back, the constant chatter in your head, the fears and phobias, the stresses and worries, the anxieties and frustrations. Anything that takes up headspace and that stops you feeling confident, calm, clear, and content.

Chapter One

Fear in Childbirth

F or both men and women, the birth of their child is one of life's magical moments. It's an experience that will stay with both of you forever, so wouldn't it be nice to approach such an experience with open hearts full of love and excitement, rather than full of fear? Unfortunately, for the majority of women of childbearing age who have not given birth, the idea of childbirth is pretty scary. It's even scary to those that HAVE given birth, especially if things didn't go too well. Sadly, in some countries where the standard of healthcare is pretty shoddy, childbirth is still responsible for a large number of fatalities. However, for the women who give birth in a developed country, the risks are very low (eight for every 100,000 births, according to the World Health Organization). So why is birth feared so much? Well, in a nutshell, it stems from a cocktail of misinformation, drama-filled TV shows and movies, relentless horror stories from friends or in the media, and a fear of the unknown.

My aim with this book to explore the fear that so often accompanies birth in an attempt to loosen its grip and change how women feel about birth. It is my hope that if more women can fear *less* when approaching their birth then we can create a ripple of positive change that goes way beyond the birthing woman. In changing birth experiences for the better, we have the potential to affect the society we live in, not only today, but far into the future. This might sound like a grand claim, but it's a fair one.

The moment of birth is a precious one, and one that needs guarding fiercely. The day a baby arrives into this world, at least three lives change forever; the mother's, the father's and the baby's. Not to mention grand-parents, siblings and other family members. When the birth is a positive and a happy one, it is a moment of pure joy. But when it isn't, it can be the stuff of nightmares.

When I say that the birthing moment goes far beyond the birthing woman, I'm referring to its impact on her baby, her partner and her immediate family. But I'm not stopping there; I'm also referring to how her experience will affect her ability to bond with her baby and her ability to parent, how it will affect her relationship with her partner, and how it might affect her mental health. It's these that affect society as a whole and birth is the common denominator. In improving birth, we have the opportunity to improve the lives of families everywhere.

So, what's fear got to do with this, and why even bother trying to banish fear from birth? When I spoke to the leading midwifery researcher, Prof. Hannah Dahlen, on my podcast she said that "Fear is the enemy of birth" and she knows what she's talking about! The most compelling reason why is that **fear directly impacts the level of pain that you will experience during childbirth**. The more fear and anxiety, the more pain. The more pain you experience, the more likely you are to make choices that may contribute or lead to a problematic, and possibly traumatic, birth. Traumatic births are known to be a contributing factor to post-natal depression, not only in women but in men too. All this is backed by research and evidence, so it's nothing new.

What is new is the arrival of some exciting and effective therapeutic techniques like Reflective Repatterning (RR), Psy-Tap, Tapas Acupressure Technique (TAT), and Havening, and their abilities to help us to free ourselves from our fears quickly and thoroughly. In taking the time to reduce your fears and anxieties before the birth, you're improving your chances of a positive birthing experience. It doesn't guarantee it, but it certainly does stack the odds in your favour.

In this book, I'm going to unravel the fears that accompany birth and then share ways that these fears can be addressed so that women (and men!) can fear **less** when it comes to birth.

The Two Types of Birth Fears

I n my experience, there are two broad categories of fear that we come across when it comes to pregnancy, childbirth, and labour:

1. Fear of the unknown

Or as I prefer to call it, *fear arising from being misinformed.*

If this is a first-time pregnancy for you, then it completely makes sense that you'll experience this fear to some degree, maybe even by the bucketload. I know I did during the early part of my first pregnancy. But a lot of this fear comes from not being well informed on matters of childbirth, and being unable to ascertain with confidence as to whether your fears are well grounded. In fact, it's likely that your fears are fed by a cocktail of seeing dramatic births on TV or in the movies, hearing your friends' horror stories, and/or seeing horrific birthing videos when you were in school (I'm sure they have ulterior motives when we are that age, so I guess it's understandable that they show us a nasty version; it certainly worked as a pretty good contraception for me).

But how much do you REALLY know about childbirth? Have you taken the time to research childbirth in any great detail in order to understand what's really going on? It's likely that if you are fearful of it, you haven't. Once we have a better understanding of the labour and childbirth process, a lot of this fear evaporates.

If, after getting your head around childbirth, you're still fearful, then what you have left is the second type of fear:

2. Deep emotional fear

This fear resides deep within your subconscious and arises from previous experiences (including those you've consciously forgotten), as well as your values and your beliefs. This kind of fear is not the type that goes away just by thinking positively or studying harder, because the rational mind is not able to change things that lie ingrained in our subconscious.

I say ingrained, because these things are. Your beliefs are rock-solid. If you have the belief that *childbirth is not natural* and the *female body is obviously not designed to have a baby's head, or body, come out of it naturally,* then being presented with solid evidence to suggest otherwise is not going to change your mind. Just as you might have the belief that you are *not good enough* or that you *always fail,* even though you hear people tell you how amazing you are and see evidence that you are perfectly capable of succeeding at things, these beliefs will dictate your thinking and your subsequent behaviour.

Fears at this level will trigger the stress response in the body, whether you like it or not. You might read about childbirth until you've devoured every book imaginable, but if when you think of [insert any aspect of childbirth here] you still can't help but feel a heavy, sick feeling in the pit of your stomach, then you have some more work to do. This feeling is hardwired in your body, at least for the time being. That doesn't mean that it can't be changed, but changing it requires a very different approach than simply *being better informed.* The thing is, fears that affect your body like this will have a magnified effect on you when you're in childbirth, which doesn't help if you're also feeling vulnerable, tired, or scared. And given that your body is the one doing all the work on the Big Day, it's better for you and baby if there aren't fears affecting it and preventing it from doing the job it is so beautifully designed to do.

This book has been written to help you to clear your fear of childbirth, whether your fears are from the first group or the second. So when it comes to helping you to become better informed, this book will only touch on what I believe are the main things that contribute to fear. However, given that what I'm trying to do here is help you clear your fears, I think it's important that you use this book as a starting point to educate yourself on childbirth. It is not a definitive guide, and there are many detailed books on childbirth out there, so please go and read them.

I want the focus of these pages to help you to clear your deep-rooted fears and prepare for a positive birth using the *Fearless Birthing* approach that I've developed as a result of the work I've done during the last seven years. It's a new approach to birth preparation that you will not have read anywhere else. I can say this with confidence because the technique that is at the heart of this approach, Reflective Repatterning, is only known by a handful of people globally and I am one of the most advanced practitioners and trainers, after its founder, Chris Milbank. As far as we are both aware, no one else has used Reflective Repatterning in this way. My first daughter was the first baby born who had been RR'd* in utero, and it was during my pregnancy with her that I developed this concept using myself as a guinea pig. With my second daughter I refined it. In between my pregnancies I shared and tested what I'd learned with pregnant friends and friends of friends.

This is how we practitioners refer to receiving Reflective Repatterning. When I first wrote this, I used the word "treated", but that made it sound like my daughter had something wrong with her, and she didn't.

Tokophobia

A book about fear of childbirth wouldn't be complete without mentioning *tokophobia*. Tokophobia is the pathological fear of pregnancy and birth that affects around 10% of women worldwide. The word comes from Greek *tokos*, meaning "childbirth," and *phobos*, meaning "fear." Phobias are a type of anxiety disorder that typically involve an intensely irrational fear of an object or situation that poses little or no danger. We often associate phobias with things like spiders or closed-in spaces.

The physical and psychological symptoms of tokophobia vary, but can include:

- Recurrent nightmares
- Hyperventilating
- Sweating and shaking
- Panic and anxiety attacks
- Crying (triggered by sight or even words)
- Nausea and vomiting
- Thoughts of death or dying

Tokophobia is classed as either primary tokophobia or secondary tokophobia. Primary tokophobia occurs in a first-time mother, who has no experience being pregnant or has not given birth before. This fear may begin well before she has reached childbearing age, perhaps when she is a child or teenager. Women who experience primary tokophobia often have a history of sexual abuse/trauma, rape, traumatic experiences of overwhelming pain, negative hospital experiences, etc. They may have been exposed to media or stories of pregnancy/birth as a horrifying and intensely painful experience, perhaps even causing death or permanent injury.

Secondary tokophobia usually occurs in women who have had prior traumatic pregnancy or birthing experiences. This trauma may relate to a negative experience with hospital staff; the feeling that they or their baby was going to die; stillbirth, late-term miscarriage, or pregnancy termination; or hyperemesis gravidarum (a debilitating form of morning sickness). One way to think about the difference between primary and secondary tokophobia is this: one is a fear arising from a *direct* experience of birth, whereas the other comes from *indirect* birth-related experiences: seeing them in films, hearing about them, or medical or sexual experiences.

However, I'd like to propose another view. Perhaps the difference between the two is that one group has a fear arising from a *conscious* memory of an experience, and the other has a fear arising from an *unconscious* memory. After all we have *all* had birth experiences - our own. Who's to say that it's not our very own arrival into the world that was traumatic and that is clouding our emotions around birth. Let's not forget, what's traumatic for one person may not be for another. A small baby who has been nurtured in their mother's womb for nine months might find all sorts trauma in things we might otherwise dismiss; being placed on a cold, metal weighing tray under bright white lights is very likely to be a horridly shocking experience for a newborn, and yet this is common practice in many hospitals.

Furthermore, there is a lot of research, as well as anecdotal evidence, to suggest that our own birth experiences affect us very deeply throughout our lives on many levels. For example, those who arrived via C-section report behavioural patterns in which they always seem to need to be pulled out of bad situations. Those that were induced early report that they never seem to feel ready for anything. We all have the experience of being born, and research tells us that if your own birth was traumatic, then you're more than likely to perpetuate that when it comes to you giving birth. One of the best ways for us to avoid repeating the pattern is to self-reflect and heal our own inner traumas, and in the case of our own entry into the world, to heal our own birth.

For me, it's not too far of a leap to suggest that primary tokophobia sufferers are simply fearful because of their own birth experience, and that it's this deeply buried trauma that's triggered by seeing births on TV or attending medical appointments. Maybe they had a traumatic hospital birth that is at the root of their fear.

When I think about my own experience of tokophobia this fits very well. When I was pregnant and tokophobic, I couldn't rid my mind of the video I saw at school of a horrible birth, and I believed this was what gave me my fear. But as I began to tackle my childbirth fears, I decided to also address any unresolved traumas that were affecting me. While I was doing some trauma clearance work on myself, I decided to work on the trauma of my own birth. At that point I didn't even *know* that I'd had a trauma, I had simply decided that *if* I had experienced trauma, then it would be cleared. If I hadn't, then I was about to waste the next fifteen minutes of my life. I was completely unprepared for what followed. In doing this trauma clearance work on myself, I hit a deep well of intense emotion that just gushed out. It took me about fifteen minutes of sobbing uncontrollably until I was able to return to a calm, still place. There were no memories as I did this, just pure emotion. Once I was able to think calmly again, I noticed how much lighter I felt. And importantly, I noticed how birth didn't make me freak out anymore. Sure, I still had fears, but these felt more surmountable now, whereas before I felt completely overwhelmed and hopeless. Now I could see a light at the end of the tunnel.

So I'd like to suggest that women with primary tokophobia, who have not yet given birth, are in fact being triggered by their own birth experience, and perhaps that is the best place for them to start in overcoming their tokophobia. Perhaps the difference between primary and secondary tokophobia is simply the difference between someone who is traumatised by a conscious memory of an experience and someone who is traumatised by an unconscious memory of an experience.

What is tokophobia like?

The first thing that strikes me is that this isn't a normal phobia in the typical sense of the word because, for one, childbirth can actually be fatal (unlike being stuck in a closed space, for example). So *irrational* is probably not the best word to use and is unfair to those who suffer from it. If you ask any woman who suffers from tokophobia, she will likely tell you that it's a rational fear that's completely understandable. For some tokophobic women, it makes complete sense. I used to be tokophobic, so I have some insight into this.

When I think about my own experience, it would fair to say that I never really thought I had this thing called tokophobia. For years I was in denial about wanting kids. On some level I knew I wanted them, but it never went any further than that. Despite being in a serious relationship, I never initiated The Kids Conversation and it never came up. To be honest, I wouldn't have even said that I had any phobia, because I wasn't being faced with the pressure of pregnancy from my friends, family, or partner. But I couldn't handle kids, especially babies. If anyone brought new babies into work for the usual "here's my new baby" drop-in session, I would run a mile. Someone tried to hand their baby over to me once and I freaked. I had to escape to the toilet and cry. I had no idea why I was crying, it just happened. I was part of a group of friends that weren't into babies and I had no family pressure to have babies, so I was able to avoid the whole baby thing quite easily, to the point that as far as I was concerned I didn't actually have a problem. If you'd asked me back then if I had tokophobia, I would have said no.

That changed the minute I discovered that I was pregnant. Then I FREAKED!! The first month of my first unplanned pregnancy was pretty dark. Adjusting to my newfound pregnant status was hard for me and my emotions were all over the place, all in shades of negative. When I miscarried at eight weeks I was relieved. Yes, I was gutted and numb with loss, but I was relieved too. That bit scared me and made me realise that something wasn't right. I thought I was a weirdo. It was then that I really started tackling my own head trash as I realised that I had just experienced something that I wasn't comfortable with: feeling relief that my baby hadn't made it.

A year later, when I became pregnant again, I was in a much better place. This time I was happy that I was pregnant. Happy, but still fearful. I had prepared myself mentally for kids, so there was less shock, but there was huge amount of fear. Fear that only showed up now that I was pregnant. I say "fear" but what I mean is "fears" with an S, because there were a ton of them. The whole idea of pregnancy freaked me out. I couldn't read about birth without crying for absolutely no reason whatsoever. In my pregnancy books, I couldn't even look at the pages that showed the birth canal. I did it once and felt a panic attack rising, so I quickly shut the book. The thought of this thing growing inside me troubled me. I kept thinking of it like a parasite feeding on its host; it was all a bit *Alien* or *X-Files*! In my first trimester, I was very clear with my birthing intentions. Plan A: drugs, lots of them. Plan B: C-section.

At that point, because I held the belief that *childbirth is painful*, I didn't realise that there was another way to do it, or that there was anything I could do about it. For me, it was about doing what I needed to do to get me through the birth. But that changed during my second trimester, when someone told me that is was possible to have a pain-free birth. It was during my quest to understand *how* a pain-free birth could be possible that I discovered the link between fear and pain during birth. This was the information I needed to propel me forward on my fear-clearance journey. Once again, I took to tackling any fear I could find relating to pregnancy and birth. By the time I reached my seventh month I was a transformed person. By month eight I ditched my plan for a hospital birth with a potential C-section as my back-up and decided for a home birth. By the time my labour came around, I was fearless and excited about the prospect of birth - a far cry from the person I had been in my first trimester.

My story ends well, because I was fortunate enough to have been introduced to a powerful therapeutic technique at the perfect time. But that's not everyone's story. Some women decide to be childless because of this fear, with some even having repeated abortions to avoid having to go through with birth. And yet there are others who are desperate to be mums and want nothing more than to have kids, but for whom the thought of having to endure nine months of hell during pregnancy and then go through with the birth is just too much to cope with. One person shared with me that she had had three abortions because of her fear of birth. Babies that she wanted. Make no mistake; this fear is a very serious one.

I now work a lot with women who have tokophobia and many of them say how important it is for them to work with someone who understands. Many healthcare professionals don't fully appreciate how tokophobia affects women and this often makes them feel isolated. It is my hope that through training other professionals in the technique that I used successfully on myself, and now others, that women with tokophobia no longer have to go through these kind of experiences.

Why Opt for a Fear-Free Birth?

S o you've picked up this book, intrigued by the idea that you can have a stress-free pregnancy and a positive, fear-free, and perhaps pain-free birth, and you're probably thinking "Crikey! That sounds like *Mission Impossible!*" Well, let me reassure you that no, it's not impossible. In fact, it's very much possible. I managed to do it (twice!) and I am not alone. One study[1] cites that 1% of women in the United States report having experienced a painless childbirth.

So why else would you bother working towards a fear-free birth?

Personal experience

Birth is momentous! It can be momentously awesome, or it can be momentously horrific and traumatic. Whichever experience you end up having, the one thing you can be sure of is this: it will have a lasting impact on you, and the experience will stay with you forever. And you will be reminded of that experience every year on poppet's birthday.

Many women describe a positive birthing experience as hugely empowering, giving them feelings of invincibility and confidence that they are able to draw on in other areas of their life. On the other hand, a negative birthing experience can weigh you down in so many ways.

By how much and for how long will depend on how bad it was and how you cope with it and heal from it. At its worse, it can lead to post-natal depression (PND) or deciding not have to any more children, which are both pretty hardcore outcomes.

I realise that just because you decide to *want* something doesn't mean you *get* it. But by making a conscious decision and setting a goal for yourself, you are already choosing a path that is more likely to bring you nearer to the outcome you desire. Unfortunately, that's not enough, especially when it comes to labour and childbirth. If you want to do a marathon, just *deciding* to do it isn't sufficient to bring you success at the finish line; you need to spend a ton of time beforehand preparing mentally and physically. And so it is with childbirth and labour. But I'm afraid to say that just because you prepare, it doesn't mean you are guaranteed to achieve your goal. Not everybody who prepares for a marathon crosses the finish line in the time they were aiming for and without injury. But they'll do infinitely better than the person who just shows up on the day expecting to get over the finish line having done diddlysquat in preparation.

Given the possible outcomes that may have arisen from me NOT taking the time to prepare for my birth - painful or traumatic birth, post-natal depression - it was an easy choice for me to take a conscious, active role in working towards my goal of having a stress-free preg-nancy and a positive, fear-free birth. But I realised *I* needed to put time and effort into this. No one else was going to do it for me; I had to step up.

Since my first pregnancy, it's struck me that many women simply don't know that there is an alternative to the dramatic, painful, or trau-matic birth. They don't realise that births can actually be calm, stress-free, exhilarating, fear-free, enjoyable, or even euphoric and orgasmic, and so they miss the opportunity to try and do something about it. But again, simply *knowing* there are alternatives doesn't necessarily mean you know HOW to go about achieving them. So that's what I want to help you to do with this book: to crank open the door and show you another path and give you a road map to help you on your way, if it's a path you want to take.

Minimise the risk of pre- and post-natal depression

No one can say for certain what causes depression in pregnancy or post-partum, and it's very likely to be as a result of a combination of factors, such as:

- Stressful and life-changing events
- Personality type
- General level of emotional resilience and "ability to cope"
- Hormones
- Pregnancy loss
- Childbirth-related distress
- Illness
- Injury or physical problems as a result of the birth
- Insufficient family or social support
- Childhood experiences of being parented
- Low self-esteem

Your birthing experience can play a role in your chances of experiencing postnatal depression. But it's also been cited that a woman's overall ability to cope with stress and emotional resilience can play a role too. So by taking a conscious and active role in reducing your levels of stress and anxiety during your pregnancy, you're maximising your chance of having a positive birthing experience, and this goes a long way in helping to reduce your chances of suffering from either post-baby blues or postnatal depression.

I think it's important to say that you can still have a positive birthing experience, even if your baby's birth doesn't go according to plan. You may well plan for a home birth or a natural birth, and for whatever reason you end up having an epidural or a C-section. This certainly doesn't mean that your birthing experience can't be a positive one. There are many women who have incredibly wonderful and positive birthing experiences like this. The important thing is HOW YOU FEEL ABOUT IT - and the great thing about that is you can influence how you feel about something. By choosing how to respond to crappy life situations, you can influence how you ultimately feel about it. The act of choosing a positive response takes you outside of a victim mentality and enables you to feel more in control of what you're feeling. This will make it easier to acknowledge negative feelings, so that you can own them, express them, and then let go of them. Better that than burying them or feeling besieged by them.

Halt genetic diseases or conditions in their tracks

Do you or members of your family suffer from genetic conditions or diseases? If you do, then you may be resigned to the fact that your baby may well end up being a sufferer too. Well, that is now known to be a flawed assumption. New discoveries in science have forced us to question what we have come to refer to as *genetic* medical conditions or diseases, the idea that if our parents have a medical condition that we are predisposed to inherit the condition or disease. Leading edge science is showing us that so-called genetic conditions are not as clear-cut as we previously thought and are not necessarily passed on to children. The field of science from which these groundbreaking ideas come is *epigenetics*. Epigenetics is the study of the environment in which the genes find themselves.

It was previously believed, and still is to a certain extent, that our DNA *controls* our biology and that once we are born with a certain gene this will control our life and health, and there is nothing we can do about it. Now we have a new field of epigenetics, the definition of *epi* being that there is something above the genes that controls how the gene is read or expressed. So what is the "above" that controls the genes? "Above" refers to the environment, which includes our emotions, beliefs, and perceptions. Dr. Bruce Lipton famously carried out some studies with stem cells to show this, and through his experiments he was able to deduce that it is the environment that the cells are in that controls how the gene is read and expressed. Put simply, we are more likely to inherit our parents' condition if we perpetuate their patterns of behaviour, emotions, thoughts, and beliefs. This is true for adopted children as well as blood children. Yes, really.

I chatted to epigeneticist Charan Surdhar on both my podcasts, *The Head Trash Show* and *Fear Free Childbirth*. During one of my chats with Charan, she talks about a piece of research that shows how some families with a history of certain types of diseases had in fact passed them onto their children. What is astounding about this research is that the children were adopted. There was no genetic link whatsoever, and yet the children still suffered from the same conditions as their parents. This suggests that it's our pattern of thoughts, beliefs, and behaviours, alongside our lifestyle choices, that have a significant impact on our health and how our body expresses certain genes.

By taking an active role in exploring our own stresses, anxieties, fears, and beliefs, we're able to change the environment that surrounds our genes. This in turn can lead to certain genes not expressing themselves in the same way they did for our parents. Or indeed, we may actually stop them from continuing to express themselves in our own bodies. This level of personal healing is widely documented and researched if you're interested in finding out more. Suffice to say, for the purposes of this book and your pregnancy, taking a conscious approach to your pregnancy is likely to benefit you and your baby's health, in ways you might not even imagine possible.

Avoid having a fussy eater

How's this for random? Not one that immediately comes to mind, but fascinating nonetheless. A recent study published in *Archives of Disease in Childhood* has shown that parental anxiety and/or depression during pregnancy is linked to a heightened risk of the child becoming a fussy eater. Now fussy kids are nothing new, and most parents put this down to it being "a phase," albeit a very annoying one. So some researchers in the Netherlands decided to try and get some answers. They examined over four thousand mother-and-child pairs, and over four thousand dads to try and understand what factors determined fussy eating in children. The health consequences for picky eaters range from constipation and weight problems to behavioural issues, so it's quite a serious issue that certainly warrants further attention.

The researchers found that maternal anxiety was directly associated with fussy eating behaviour by the time their child was 4 years old and this was irrespective of their own symptoms when the child was 3. Apparently, the more anxious the mothers felt, the fussier the child.

They go on to say that the mum's antenatal symptoms predicted a four-year-old's fussy eating behaviour, irrespective of whether she had symptoms when the child was three and that this "strongly suggests that the direction of the associations with mothers' antenatal symptoms is from mother to child. . . . Clinicians should be aware that not only severe anxiety and depression, but also milder forms of internalising problems can affect child eating behaviour."

Now, I don't know what it's like to have a fussy eater, because both my kiddies eat absolutely everything (maybe because of my obsession with obliterating my stresses!), but I can only imagine how difficult it would make parenting. Given the importance of food and a healthy diet, this is yet another compelling reason to *do the work* and put in the effort now that will reap you dividends later.

Chapter Two

Fearless Birthing

I could say that Fearless Birthing is *just* a birth preparation approach, but in fact it's so much more than that. To experience a truly fearless birth requires you to have faced your fears and made peace with them. But I'm not just talking about birthing fears - I'm talking life fears! This includes all sorts: relationship fears, health fears, parenting fears, work fears, sex fears, friendship fears . . . the list goes on.

Among professional birthing companions, such as midwives and doulas, birth is often considered to be microcosm of life, and our birthing journey is a reflection of our struggles with ourselves and the people around us. The sheer power of birth magnifies and shines a light on all those aspects of ourselves. Add to that the immenseness of this momentous transitional moment and you have the potential for a high pressure or stressful event, particularly if the mother has lots of unresolved fears and anxieties with herself, her partner, her relation-ship or her ideas of motherhood. These often rear their ugly head during the transition phase of birth. So when I'm talking about Fearless Birthing being much bigger than simply a birth preparation approach, it's because it has the potential to be truly transformational for the mother who takes her Fearless Birthing mission seriously. I did, and it was.

During my first pregnancy I was a stressy, fearful thing who was a bit all over the place. I was grateful to have recently discovered and trained in the therapy Reflective Repatterning, because it was finally helping me to sort my head out. Up until that point I had tried a ton of different things with limited success; trying to sort my head out was not a new mission.

But pregnancy forced my hand. I now had a focus for me to sort my head out - and an immovable deadline! Not only was I conscious that I needed to make the mental and emotional shift from childless and free to mother, but I also had to deal with the birthing fears that were crippling me. Discovering early on in my pregnancy the link between fear and pain in childbirth was the piece that finally helped me figure out a way forward, especially as I'd just learned a powerful fear-clearance technique. It was like the gods had come together to help me.

I focussed ruthlessly on clearing my birthing fears because I was terrified more than anything of the PAIN! And if clearing my fears meant I could avoid pain during birth, then I was happy to sign up. But I never for one minute realised how far-reaching this would be for me personally. When I start doing something, I'm like a dog with a bone, and I approached this with the same kind of efficiency as I would approach a work project. When it came to me trying to pin down what my fears were, I didn't stop at my birthing fears. I went all the way and lifted the lid on all of them! My fear of being a mother - would I be any good? My fear of being able to keep my relationship together (my parents divorced when I was four, so understandable, I guess). My fear of being able to love my body again; my fears of dying . . . well, you get the picture!

Looking back, it's pretty obvious that doing this kind of work would be transformational. If you're going to make peace with as many of your major life fears as you can, of course it's going to make a difference. But not many people choose to do this kind of work. Many would LIKE to, but don't know how - they don't have the expertise or the tools. And then there are those who don't have the heart or the ovaries for it. For some it feels like opening Pandora's box and that can seem scary. But what's on the other side is so, so worth it.

So what was on the other side for me? Well, the thing I wanted! The reason I did it all in the first place: a beautiful, positive birthing experience. As a bonus it was also natural and painless. And when the time came for me to do it again, it was even better; as well as being painless, my second birth was euphoric too. Utter magic! But let's just park the births for a minute. What else?

Well, I was calmer, much calmer. In fact, late on during my pregnancy I was so calm, I was constantly having people tell me how calm I looked and how they'd never seen a heavily pregnant women look so calm before. This calmness stayed with me into motherhood. Despite being challenging, my first few weeks as a new mother didn't completely freak me out. Sure I struggled with the newness of it all, the lack of sleep in the first two months, but on the whole my first few months as a mum were lovely. I didn't feel anxious from not knowing what the hell was going on. I didn't feel stressed from feeling out of my depth. I was able to focus on being present with my baby and tuning in to her needs and I didn't find it a struggle. It felt natural and do-able. My journey into motherhood didn't feel like a bumpy crash-landing into chaos, but more like a controlled, smooth screech into stillness. This was a big deal. I used to be this stressy-anxious thing who looked like a rabbit in headlights most of the time. But now I wasn't, AND I was new mum!

Is clearing fears a good thing?

Whenever there's discussion around the idea of clearing or overcoming our fears, there are always a bunch of people that jump up to remind us that our fears are good, and I completely agree with them. If it wasn't for mine, I wouldn't have stepped up. But before we start finding brilliant excuses for not bothering with this important work, I think it's key for us to understand the distinction between fear that is a *normal emotional response*, and a *deep-rooted* or *irrational* fear. So what's the difference?

The difference between the two comes down to this: a normal emotional response is one that is triggered by some kind of environmental trigger or situation, and once the trigger or situation has passed, so does the fear. When you're approaching the edge of a cliff, your fear warns you to stay away from the edge. But once you're back in town, you're not constantly in fear of "the edge"; you've forgotten about it and your fear has passed. The emotional signal from your body is no longer required. A deep-rooted or irrational fear is a lurker. It stays with you and can be easily triggered by something as simple as merely thinking about it (creating it in your mind) or environmental factors that might be slightly similar or slightly related to THE THING. For example, if you're on a bus and are reminded about your fear of "the edge" and you feel the fear come over you when you get to the edge of the pavement or you see a poster of someone bungee jumping off a ledge. This isn't a healthy emotional response because at that moment in time, your life isn't in actual danger, so there is no need for you to experience fear.

When I talk about clearing fears, I'm referring to those pesky deep-rooted ones that lurk unhelpfully beneath the surface, interfering in the day-to-day when they're simply not required. What I'm not talking about is clearing the fears that help you to survive or cope with everyday life. Fears are good and we need them. But we don't need to be carrying more than we need, because they'll just weigh us down. These are the ones we need to relieve ourselves of. We need to restore our emotional settings to default. It's like with your phone or you computer. You've got old apps that you used to use, but not anymore and after a while it becomes slow and sluggish. They've left traces of *stuff* that create glitches and bugs. Sometimes we just need to *reset to factory settings*. That's what I'm talking about here . . . getting rid of the emotional stuff that no longer serves you and is weighing you down.

I would also like to emphasise that when I talk about Fearless Birthing, I'm referring to you being fearless *while* birthing, not all the time. I'm not in any way saying that we should banish fear from our lives. Fears are a good thing and they serve us well, but not while we're in labour. When I'm birthing a baby, I want to be fearless; I don't want fears interfering with my mind and my body. I want you to fear *less* when it comes to your up-coming birth.

Making peace with our fears

I think it would be fair to say that most people fear their fears. They don't like them and they probably avoid them. I'd like to suggest instead that we make peace with our fears and embrace them; to love them and appreciate them. Our fears desperately want to help us; they have our survival in mind. They're just a tad confused. So we need to treat them with kindness and embrace them. We might not be delighted at their presence, but we can at least be tolerant and understanding of them. I love how Elizabeth Gilbert refers to fear in her book Big Magic: "Sure you can invite fear along for the ride, but it's got to sit in the backseat and it has no say on the route, the music, or the snacks!" I think this captures the essence of making peace with your fear perfectly.

In doing this we're better able to understand them and the intention that lies behind them. Often, our fears hold gifts for us, but only if we're open to them. We might break through a new door that we had previously kept tightly shut. We have the potential to reveal new parts of ourselves. We have the possibility of growing stronger. What's not to like about fears?

Conscious mama with courage!

The mama that chooses to embark on a Fearless Birthing journey is a courageous one. Taking a look in the mirror and facing your fears requires courage. Which, by the way, is a great quality for a mama to have! So if a mama decides to use her precious pregnancy to embark on this journey she should be applauded and supported. More of us need to be doing this, because if we did the world would be a better place. A woman that chooses to be conscious during her pregnancy in this way is already showing us what a great mother she will be.

We all know that we get our emotional crap from our parents, right? All our quirks and foibles, our character faults and issues. At one time in our lives, we've all dumped them firmly at our parents' door when it comes to blame. And rightly so. The psychologists agree too. Our family patterns of behaviour perpetuate themselves unless some self-reflection and healing takes place. So when a mother is consciously taking steps to take a closer look at her own personal fears and anxieties, she's raising her level of self awareness in such a way that she's already doing something to stop her crap from being passed on to her children. Of course, there's no guarantee because this kind of work never ends. This level of self-awareness, self-examination, and healing needs to be maintained. So if you're a mama-to-be reading this and silently committing to this journey in your mind I salute you. You have my utmost respect and admiration!

Transformational you say?

For many, the idea of taking a look in the mirror feels overwhelming. It's much easier to avoid it and instead fill our lives with distractions. Meanwhile, our stress levels get more out of control and we counter it with even more food, drink, shopping, spending, or whatever it takes to distract us from the emotional craziness that rules the inside of our heads. In clearing our fears and our stresses, we too experience a birth: a re-birth. In stripping away our fears and stresses, we reveal new aspects of ourselves. In fact, what is really happening is that we're becoming a more concentrated version of ourselves, less diluted with all the crap. Through undertaking the Fearless Birthing journey, this new, authentic woman is more connected to her essence, and she is grounded, sure of her very nature and able to trust her instincts. It's with this gentle strength that she is able to offer herself, her child, and her family pure, unconditional love and compassion in abundance.

The positive childbirth experience that can await you at the end of your Fearless Birthing journey can empower you and give you the strength and confidence to be who you want and need to be, for yourself, for your partner, and for your children.

Fearless Birthing helps to bring all this about. But it doesn't just end when poppet is born. All the preparation work you put in stays with you. Your ability to manage fear stays with you, as does your ability to remain calm in the face of pressure - something you will need an unlimited supply of as a parent.

What if the sh*t hits the fan during birth? Then what?

Birth is unpredictable. We hear this all the time. Well, yes it is. But not really. There are only so many ways birth can happen and it's all been seen before. It's not that unpredictable. In preparing for birth, there is nothing stopping you from preparing emotionally for various outcomes, including those you DEFINITELY DON'T WANT. When you make peace with these unwanted outcomes, if they should present themselves, you'll be much less likely to work yourself into a fearful, stressed-out frenzy. Approaching birth fearlessly means that even if things don't go as planned, you are able to respond calmly and flexibly. If you are confronted with decisions you need to make during the course of your labour and childbirth, you will be in a much better place to be able to respond calmly, rather from a place of fear and stress, which means you're more likely to make a decision you're happy with later. It's the rushed decisions made in fear that can contribute to negative birthing experiences. Fear is never a good place to be making important decisions from.

My ultimate goal for the Fearless Birthing journey is this: a positive birthing experience whichever way it unfolds on the day, and that your birthing experience continues to bring you joy every time your baby has a birthday. Even if things didn't go the way you want, if you're comfortable with how things unfolded and can look back on your experience with joy, then that is THE MOST IMPORTANT THING. The goal isn't a natural birth, or a home birth, or a water birth. It is entirely possible to have a traumatic water birth, and who'd want that? No, a positive birthing experience is the Holy Grail. Yes, beyond that we can strive for natural or whatever. But for our future emotional well-being we need to feel positively about our experience. This is why it's so important to prepare yourself emotionally.

What about hypnobirthing?

You might be wondering "Hey Lex! Why didn't you just do some hypnobirthing? Surely that's what you needed to prepare for birth?" Well I did! When I was pregnant and fearful, the first glimmer of hope that came my way was when I discovered hypnobirthing and the link between fear and pain. I have a lot to thank hypnobirthing for. It was responsible for introducing me to the birth education that would give me my "aha" moment. But for me, it only took me so far. Despite reading many of the books and listening to more than my fair share of hypnobirthing tracks, I was still stuck with my fear. To be honest, I think it started to unravel for me with the hypnobirthing tracks; they really annoyed me. Don't get me wrong. I love a bit of woo - as a therapist, my tools of choice are energy therapies - so I can woo with the best of them. I just couldn't bear those new-agey guided meditations walking through meadows or sandy beaches that I kept coming across. And I really struggled with imagining my vagina as a flower. The more I got into hypnobirthing, the more I kept stumbling across elements of it that just weren't working for me. I found this hugely frustrating because deep down I knew that I really needed what hypnobirthing was offering.

One of my big gripes was how I was being discouraged from using certain words. The word "pain" is pretty much banned in hypnobirthing circles, while the word "contractions" is switched for "surges". This doesn't sit well with me at all. It's all very well deciding that you're going to stop using these words, but how on earth are you going to get everyone else to stop using them? The thought of having to tell my care providers that they can't use the word "pain" in my presence is just plain ridiculous. I'm of the opinion that if you try and change the world around you, you're in for a long, hard slog. It's much easier to change yourself. So, if you have a problem with the word pain, then change how you FEEL about it so that it's no longer a problem for you.

What kind of message are you sending when you ask people to change their behaviour in your presence? I felt like it either made me sound like I'm high maintenance or that I had sensitivities and that they needed to pussyfoot around me. Neither of those sound like someone who's sure of herself, do they? Don't get me wrong, I think hypnobirthing works brilliantly for many women, but it's not for everyone. I realised that I needed something quite different. I also needed something that was going to clear my fears. And that's when it hit me; I should try using this new therapy I'd just been trained in, Reflective Repatterning. Apparently it ate fears for breakfast, so what was I waiting for? So I decided to come up with my own version of hypnobirthing but without the hypnosis, and without the annoying tracks. And where I get to use whatever language I want. The more I gave this serious thought, the more I realised that Reflective Repatterning was a great candidate for the job. But before I could crack on I had to tinker with it so I could use it on myself and be my own therapist. There were only a handful of us trained at this point and I sure as hell couldn't afford private sessions - not with my list of fears! I needed an easy to use DIY version. So, that became my new task.

What is Reflective Repatterning?

R eflective Repatterning is a new therapeutic technique from the field of Energy Psychology (EP) that was created by Chris Milbank. Milbank is known for his innovative approaches in the therapy world, and in addition to being trained to an advanced level in many mind and body therapies, he has also worked closely with many of the leading figures in modern therapy, most notably Roger Callahan, who created Thought Field Therapy (TFT).

Its name is a good place to start as it can help us to understand more about what it is and how we can use it. On one hand, *reflective* hints at the fact that it forces us to take a look at ourselves and *reflect* on who we are, how and what we think, and why we behave the way we do. But the truth is, *reflective* reveals the significance that the universal law of opposites (AKA the law of polarity) plays in our emotions, values, and beliefs. In fact, this universal law is so important that it forms part of the very DNA of Reflective Repatterning and informs its whole approach. It's this very aspect that enables Reflective Repatterning to be combined with many other therapeutic techniques to turbo-power their effectiveness. Reflective Repatterning works brilliantly when paired with techniques such as Neuro-Linguistic Programming (NLP), Thought Field Therapy (TFT), Emotional

Freedom Technique (EFT), and Havening. It can also be used in tandem with many body therapies.

Repatterning refers to its ability to re-pattern our thoughts and behaviours. Quite remarkably, Reflective Repatterning is able to quickly neutralise our negative thoughts, feelings, emotions, and limiting beliefs, thereby offering us more freedom, choice, and flexibility in how we think, feel, and behave. *Neutralise* might sound like a bit of a hardcore term, but it's not - it's just a great way of describing what's going on. Let's take a quick look at what Google says about the word: *neutralise: make (something) ineffective by applying an opposite force or effect.* You see? It's the law of opposites making another appearance. By applying an equal but opposite force, the thing in question is neutralised. So when we're talking about emotions, we're simply neutralising the negative emotions using opposing forces to give us new ways of thinking, feeling, and behaving.

When I first used Reflective Repatterning, I found it quite incredible. When I would talk about it to friends, I described the feeling as being like "having my head trash cleared away," like one minute my head was full of crap, and in the next it was gone. On many occasions I couldn't even remember what I was so bothered about before, like there was no trace of it. It was this feeling that inspired the term *head trash* for me and *head trash clearance.* That's how it felt! I'm not laying claim to that term, it just felt like a perfect way to describe my experience. I was one of the first people to be trained in this therapy, and I was fortunate to work alongside Milbank for a number of years as he was developing it. During that time we trained many other therapists, counsellors and coaches and I remember being constantly amazed at the level of change we'd witness in our students, and hearing their stories of successes with their clients.

Why Reflective Repatterning is ideal for clearing pregnancy fears

There are many tools and techniques that can help to reduce our fears and clear our negative emotions, however, many of these work mainly with the mind. The thing is, clearing fears from the mind is only doing half the job; we need to clear this emotional energy from our body too, and that's what Reflective Repatterning is able to do so brilliantly. This is partly due to the fact that it's an Energy Psychology (EP) technique. EP techniques work with the energy system, which is the interface between mind and body. In working with the energy system, we're able to clear out our mind AND body, which makes any clearance work much more effective because it's working more deeply and thoroughly.

Clearing negative emotions from our mind AND body is particularly relevant when it comes to pregnancy and childbirth because of the emotional and physical nature of birth. As a pregnant woman, you don't want any negative emotions in your mind or your body. So much will be demanded of your mind and body as you go through pregnancy and childbirth that you simply do not want any part of your system being clogged up in that way, preventing nature from doing what nature does best. Imagine you're about to have a Pap smear test. As you think about that, what do you notice in your body? (If you're a man reading this - imagine watching a high-speed cricket ball heading towards your balls - what do you notice?). It's probable that your legs tensed for a flashing moment and you might even feel the need to cross your legs. That was negative emotional energy showing up in your body creating tension. Very often emotions get trapped in our bodies and can manifest in things like tension headaches or backaches. This is NOT something you want to encourage when it comes to birth, especially if you have a fear of birth that makes you want to tighten or cross your legs. Imagine how that would affect your ability to birth your baby. For me, this is why energy psychology therapies are perfect companions to help you prepare for birth and to use during birth.

What is Fearless Birthing?

F earless Birthing is a birth prep approach where the absolute focus is on taking you from fearful to fearless, with a very clear goal for you; to have a positive birth experience. So naturally it includes fear-clearance at its core, but it also includes other aspects that we know can help you prepare for your birth.

Preparing for your birth, can feel like a bit of a mountain to climb. It's a pretty unique scenario that combines mental, emotional and physical preparation with learning loads of new stuff, some of which might be completely alien to you (biology, parenting, science etc). On top of all that, it culminates in a life-defining event that you can't escape from and that you probably won't even have the chance to decide when it happens. You'll just have to wait for it to arrive in its own time. It's no surprise that many women choose to opt-out of all this and just bury their heads in the sand until the last minute.

But, *winging it* or *going with the flow* is NOT an option if you're serious about wanting a positive birth. Did you know that women who wing it are more likely to end up with the kind of birth a super fearful woman has. i.e. - long labour, painful, probably medicalised and with a high chance of emergency c-section. In other words, a challenging if not difficult birth experience, that could leave you traumatised. Why risk it? Much better to prepare. The thing is preparing effectively for your birthing experience involves a lot more than simply clearing your fears.

The Fearless Birth Prep Road Map

Here are what I believe are the essential steps that will lead you to your fearless birth.

1. Identify the birth you want

This might sound obvious but it's important. With anything in life, if you want to achieve your goal, you have to be clear on the goal you're aiming for and birth is no different. Of course, just because you've identified it, doesn't mean you'll get it, but it will definitely increase your chances. Do your research and think about what you want.

2. Identify your fears and stresses

As you think about your birth right now, what fears are you aware of? Perhaps you don't have any. Early on in pregnancies, this is possible but it may well be because you're not fully aware of them yet. If you're feeling confident and excited, that's brilliant. But don't make the mistake of thinking that you don't have any. Be open to explore this as soon as possible.

It's important to understand what your fears and stresses are. The techniques that I've brought together for Fearless Birthing require you to address specifics. It's hard to work on clearing your to-do list if you've never taken the time to *write* your to-do list. Same goes for this. There's an additional benefit to this aspect, though, and it's this: just the act of thinking through your "stuff" (head trash, issues, life challenges, stresses, etc.) starts a very important process of raising your self-awareness. Having dedicated thinking time to figuring out all that stuff whirling round in your head can help you to calm it all down a bit. Often our chaotic headspace is simply a result of hiding from it all, or denying it.

Have you ever had a pile of clothes that built up on a chair or on the floor in a corner of the room? Eventually it starts to weigh you down seeing that mess. You might even be tempted to shove everything into the bottom of the closet just to get it out of the way. But even if you do, in your head you *know* there's a crappy mess at the bottom of your closet and it will niggle you every time you open it. If you took the time to go through the clothes then you'd feel much better, and in the process you'd probably spot things that you can get rid of, or can put in the wash. Even if you just left the folded clothes in a pile on the chair, you'd still *feel* better about it and would find it much easier to go on to the next step of having a proper tidy-up. It's all about the baby steps!

Taking the time to THINK your head trash through is valuable to the whole process. Often our fears and anxieties seem really overwhelming, but once you take the time to figure out what they actually are, the overwhelming-ness of it all starts dissolving and it starts to seem much more manageable.

3. Educate yourself about birth

If it's your first time, then it's important to educate yourself as much as possible so that you're prepared. We can't guarantee any outcome when it comes to birth, but being informed will help you to cope much better and feel less fearful. You will be faced with many decisions during your pregnancy and birth, some which carry important consequences.

Being able to make a decision from an informed place will ensure that you're more likely to be happy with your decisions later. No one wants to be thinking "*I wish I'd done my homework*" after the difficult birth that affected you badly. And many do!

* * *

These first three steps don't necessarily have to come in the order I've written. It may well be that you need to educate yourself BEFORE you can identify your ideal birth. Perhaps you identify your birth, then educate yourself on it and refine your ideal birth based on what you've learned. Or maybe you can't identify your birth because your fears dominate. If that's you, start by figuring what your fears are, educate yourself on those aspects and then identify your ideal birth.

4. Birth Planning

This is where you make the subtle transition from *imagining* your ideal or perfect birth, to some focused thinking about the practicalities. This is where your birth starts taking shape and goes further than simply deciding whether you want a hospital or a home birth, or whether you want the water birth or the epidural. At this stage you'll start pulling together your birth preferences or birth plan document.

5. Boost your birth confidence

No matter how you feel about birth, feeling even MORE confident about it can only help. Your level of confidence going into your birth is crucial, so finding ways to boost your birth confidence is an important step. This will differ for everyone but might include things like listening to positive birth stories, stopping listening to scary ones and people who aren't supportive or encouraging, and posting positive birthing affirmations around your home.

6. Clearance time

If you've followed the steps already, then everything you've done so far will have reduced any fear you might have by quite a bit, so any fears that are still lurking at this stage will need some focused clearance action.

There are three ways you can do the clearance work:

1. You can do it yourself (using this book)
2. You can work with a Fearless Birthing Practitioner privately (or therapist or a practitioner of another emotional clearance technique).
3. You can listen to one of my Fearless Birthing Meditations. (I've created a number of these to tackle the most common birthing fears)

You keep on clearing until you've worked through your list and until you're in place where you feel completely calm and positive about your upcoming birth.

7. Prepare for the birth you DON'T want
This might sound silly and counter-intuitive but it's worth doing. Just because you want a home birth, doesn't mean you'll get it. Just because you want the hospital birth, doesn't mean you'll get it. You might have a planned c-section but go into labour before hand... birth is unpredictable! The best way to ensure that you feel as calm and as confident as you can is to be ready for all outcomes. When you're in labour, if things go off plan and you get frazzled, your frazzled-ness will affect the birth negatively. If you're prepared for all possible outcomes - especially the one you really DON'T want - then you'll be better able to cope if things go off plan, which ultimately is better for your birth.

8. Prepare for the birth you DO want
Of course you need to do this! Preparing for birth is crucial, and it will include things like doing the practical preparation as well as mental, physical and emotional preparation. I'll talk more about this later on but this is pretty much what this whole book is about. Having said that, being mindful and deliberate about the birth you want is what this is about.

9. Practise managing your mindset for birth

One thing that will help you to boost your confidence going into your birth is having a bunch of tools you can use to help you cope with what's happening. The thing is, you will need time to practise using these tools and techniques so that you feel confident using them. They need to be second nature to you on the day so time spent practising is worth it.

Throughout the rest of this book I'm going to dive into some of these into quite some depth, but not all of them, otherwise this would be a tome. A huge part of preparing for your birth is learning about birth and there are plenty of brilliant books that can help you with that. You also need to learn about the choices and risks that you face and this will mean speaking to your care providers and carrying out your own research.

Over the course of this book, I will be focussing on the mindset elements of this road map; the emotional and the mental.

Bonus Content

Do you want help preparing for your birth?

I've created a free 5-day email challenge to get you started. Once you sign up you will receive a daily email which will help you to think things through and prepare for your birth.

Sign up for the *Fearless Birth Prep Challenge* here: www.fearfreechildbirth.com/fearless-birth-prep-challenge/

Dana's Fearless Birthing Story

I t's all very well, me wittering on about my journey but I don't want you thinking that I'm this special snowflake. This approach is already helping other women to experience their positive births. So before I carry on, I'd like to share Dana's account of her Fearless Birthing experience.

I will do my best to articulate the profound effect your head trash clearance method had on my pregnancy.

About 6 years ago I thought an elective c-section was the way to go. I am the biggest wimp when it pertains to pain and I didn't think I could cope with a natural birth.

Over the past 4 years I have really enveloped myself into the health & wellness world and I learned how incredibly impactful the birthing process is to a child's lifelong health. Once I understood this and the true consequences of a c-section birth I wanted to avoid it. However, I still didn't know how to manage the pain. Then I found your podcast & head trash clearance method.

Your podcast opened my eyes up to an entirely new way to view natural birth. It's the first time I saw birth as a manageable and even enjoyable experience. Instead of seeing birth as an automatic painful experience, I saw it's potential. That it could be enjoyable, intense, maybe painful but overall life changing if I surrendered to it and relaxed into the experience.

In spite of having a new view of birth, that didn't change that I still had underlying and deep rooted fears. I feared I couldn't cope with the intensity, I feared I wouldn't have the stamina needed for birth, I feared I would let my husband and our daughter down, that I would lose control of my emotions and become frantic, that I would end up with a c-section or something would happen to our daughter. This is where the head trash method saved the day.

Using the method laid out in your videos I began working through each fear. By the time I was done working through them I no longer felt this deep rooted fear that engulfed my mind and body. Instead I felt light. I could acknowledge the previous fear without any associated emotion. It became the same as making any generic statement such as "I'm going to wear white socks today".

What's even better is that I didn't have to set aside hours upon hours to work through my fears. When a fear popped up during my pregnancy I spent about 5-10mins using the head trash clearance method & the fear was gone. It was incredibly empowering to know I could successfully rid myself of a fear in such a short period of time.

As my birth approached I felt at peace and excited to meet my daughter. With my fears cleared I knew I could handle anything that came my way.

My birth was incredible. Challenging? Definitely. But full of love. I never had an ounce of fear the entire time. I was able to completely relax into every contraction and every stage. I progressed quickly and after 7 hours of active labour, including 12 minutes of pushing, I had the most beautiful baby girl in my arms. Not bad for a first time mama who once wanted to have an elective c-section!

Once more I was so proud of myself for embracing every moment of my daughters birth. I never got snarky with my husband or anyone else. I only used a little bit of gas during transition. I focused on breathing my way through the labour, taking one breath at a time. And believe it or not, I look forward to doing it again!

The head trash clearance method was pivotal in allowing me to have such an incredible birth. It allowed me to give myself and my daughter the type of birth I dreamed of and I am eternally grateful.

Chapter Three

The Consciousness of Pregnancy

Y ou will often hear how magical a time pregnancy can be, and yes, I agree it can be. But it can also be horrid, and everything else in between. My first pregnancy was a delightful breeze. I escaped the hormonal rollercoaster of the first trimester and was blessed with only intense feelings of tiredness (and of course my fear!). But even then they were nothing like my second pregnancy. I had no morning sickness or other annoying pregnancy symptoms. All in all, I felt like I was taking it in stride. I was always being told that I was glowing and how well pregnancy seemed to suit me. This pregnant glow stayed with me until the birth and was nothing like my second pregnancy, which, looking back, felt like a polar opposite.

My second pregnancy was a complete nightmare, at least for me. Putting my geriatric age aside, one thing I'm sure of today is that there is no way I'd contemplate having another child. And that's not because I couldn't face going through birth again, it's because I couldn't face the prospect of being pregnant and risk going through anything like my last pregnancy; it felt like this never-ending barrage of relentless, unpleasant emotions and physical symptoms. My first trimester was a depressing combination of horrific hormones, dark emotions, and deeply intense fatigue and exhaustion that never seemed to go away.

The tiredness of my first pregnancy was nothing compared to how I felt throughout my second pregnancy. Most of my weekends went like this: I would rise on a Saturday, eat breakfast, and have to go back to bed because I couldn't stay upright. After about two hours of sleep, I'd have no energy to get up and would have to text my partner to bring me some food in bed - usually a banana - just so I could have the energy to get out of bed. I'd get up to have some lunch and then have to go back to bed, again, because I could barely stay upright. I'd sleep for a couple of hours and then repeat the banana request until I could get up from bed. Then I'd have dinner, put my daughter to bed, and go back to bed. What kind of craziness is that?

I quickly learned that the little thing that was growing inside of me needed a lot more energy than my first daughter. I had to honour her demands and increase my food and energy intake, as well as take more rest, just so I could get through the day. I would often get caught out with the tiredness thing, but when I remembered that it might be lack of energy, it was quickly sorted out by eating more food. This extreme hunger that my unborn baby had is actually just who she is. At the time, I thought I was carrying a boy, not a girl! When I was breastfeeding, she was relentless in her appetite and even now she eats crazy quantities, which I don't even know where she puts it - her appetite exceeds her big sister sometimes. My need to slow down really affected me in a bad way at first. I was used to doing stuff and not lazing around, so this exhaustion really played into my feelings about how useless I felt.

Hormones are notorious for wreaking havoc on your emotional state, and one thing I learned during this pregnancy is that they magnify the emotions that are already there. So if you're feeling in the slightest way delicate, then by the time your hormones have finished with you, you'll be a complete emotional wreck. Yes, that was me. With bells on!

In the intervening years since having my first daughter, I continued my personal head trash clearance work. My first pregnancy showed me how powerful and transformational head trash clearance was, and I wanted to continue.

The thing about head trash is that it's just like normal trash: it's made up of stuff that you used to want or need, but that is no longer needed or clutters your space. The other similarity with normal trash is that there is constantly new trash to get rid of. You never get to pause and say, "That's it! I've finished clearing out my rubbish. No more rubbish clearance for me!" Before long, you'll go out and acquire something else, then you'll use or consume it, and then there'll be something else to get rid of, either the packaging or remnants of the thing itself. It's a never-ending cycle of clearance.

Our head trash is just like that, which is one of the reasons that I love it as a term for all that stuff that takes up headspace. Much of our head trash as adults is the remnants of behavioural or emotional habits from our childhood and growing up. As children, we absorb beliefs and emotional habits from our parents without necessarily choosing them. Perhaps they served us well back then, but maybe less so now. The thing is, we still hold on to them when in fact they're just surplus to requirements. What we really need is a clear-out; a head trash clear-out.

The other main reason I like the term "head trash" is that it's neutral and doesn't carry any inherent meaning, other than "no longer needed" or "surplus to requirements." It's not *good* or *bad*, and so it holds us back from judging it. We don't judge our household rubbish, we simply accept it for what it is and get rid of it. Many therapists typically will ask you what *issue* or *problem* you want help with. These words bring with them judgement and opinions that can cloud our thinking. "Problem" or "issue" makes it sound like a bad thing, or something we should be ashamed of it. If we're wrestling with stuff, the last thing we need is to feel like we have this bad, problematic stuff to be ashamed of. It may well be the case, but we don't need to ram it home so forcefully through poor use of language.

If we were children when we decided that we needed to be selfish to survive our emotionally abusive parents, being selfish back then was a good thing that helped us to survive. Selfishness can be a good thing, even as an adult. Selfishness isn't bad or good, it just is. But perhaps we're being too selfish; we have it out of balance. So thinking about our selfishness as a bad thing isn't helpful, because in many ways it's a good thing: it's served us well. We just need to get rid of the excess selfishness that exists within us, not all of it. Big difference.

Are you a hoarder? Some people hate getting rid of stuff. I used to be that person, keeping all sorts of crap just in case I might need it some day. This is a pattern that also applies to head trash. Many people can't face the prospect of letting go of their head trash and will make a ton of excuses to avoid doing so. Usually there's a secondary gain to them having this stuff, the most popular being that they receive love from and/or a connection with others by having this thing. For example, someone who is depressed might have family members frequently popping in to visit them or bring them food. Perhaps they feel that if they weren't depressed, their family wouldn't visit so much, and they fear being lonely or having to go out and make friends. Other people feel weird about the possibility of letting go of this thing, given that they've been affected by it for so long in their life and in some way it's part of their identity; if they get rid of it, what will that mean in terms of who they are? Head trash can be comforting, and as we're creatures of habit, we hold onto it because it's what we know and we're afraid of change: "Yes, things might be shit now. But if I change, what if they become more shit? I can't risk my life being even more shit, so I'll just stay in this pile of shit, that I know and have gotten used to."

In the first trimester of my second pregnancy, I was struggling big time. The combination of hormones and difficult emotions made for a horrid cocktail. I felt like I was completely useless, and I couldn't face the world. I'd sit at my desk in tears, thinking how utterly crap I was at my work. I was meant to be launching a new aspect to the business that involved making sales calls and getting meetings. This was not a good headspace to be in. Feeling crap about who you are and what you do does not make a great sales call. So I procrastinated. I procrastinated by slumping into a crying mess at my desk. Given the therapies and techniques that I'm familiar with, I was always trying to figure out what on earth was going on in my head so that I could get to the bottom of it and move on. Instead of working on my business, I would spend days throwing every technique I knew at myself to try and sort out the mess in my head.

When nothing worked I came to a huge realisation: *this isn't me.* All these feelings weren't me, they just happened to be passing through my mind. This was purely a hormonal experience and I needed to avoid grabbing hold of these feelings as if they were mine. In fact, I just needed to keep my head down, hold tight, and ride the emotional wave. As long as I kept my head above water, I'd be OK.

For me, keeping my head above water meant earning money. And as I was clearly in no fit state to run my business, I decided to put it on hold and look for a contract job doing what I used to do before changing careers. I needed something I could do on autopilot with minimal effort, something that didn't require me to feel confident to achieve results. It was really hard to make the decision to put my business on hold because I'd put so much into it. But I had to face reality that while my emotions were tangled in a downward spiral, I had to put it on hold. Despite being very difficult to digest, this realisation was enlightening for me. Realising that these feelings occupying my headspace weren't me, just chemicals, was hugely liberating. It meant that I could just sit with them and not jump into them.

When I learned how to meditate at my local Buddhist centre, one thing they taught us was this: "Just imagine your thoughts being clouds that pass through the sky in your mind. Notice them and let them pass, just don't jump onto them." This really helped me to grasp the idea of meditation, but it lacked something for me, so I tweaked it to make more sense; to me it felt more like being on a train platform and watching the trains pass through. My thoughts and feelings back then felt like big, noisy (and slightly scary) fast-moving trains. Not slow, drifting, white fluffy clouds. And anyway, I'd never contemplate jumping on a cloud, but trains? Yes. The idea of being on a train platform and just letting the trains pass through without getting distracted by where they were going and whether or not I wanted to get on them was something I could relate to. Sitting on a train platform when you can hear a big, noisy freight train approaching in the distance is how I felt sometimes. Sitting still and letting the all-consuming, shuddering, ear-deafening sound of carriage after carriage trample over me until it pummelled its way into the distance. Before my realisation, I would've leapt on to that crazy, noisy ride believing that it was for me, and I would have let it drag me to wherever it was going, whether I wanted to go there or not. Now I could just let it pass and calmly sit still, without feeling its pull.

During my monthly menstrual cycle, there is always one day in which I feel completely useless, teary, and depressed. On that particular day everything looks dark and depressing: my decisions, my relationships, my work, and my life. It always catches me off guard and sucks me in. You'd think I would've figured it out by now and know what's happening, but I haven't and I fall for it every. single. time! My first trimester was like that, but for weeks on end. If I hadn't been able to make that shift from feeling like those emotions *were* me to feeling them just passing through me, I think I would've fallen head-first into an extended bout of prenatal depression. I'm pretty sure I was there for a brief time, but I managed to escape. If I didn't have my toolbox of techniques and therapies that I trusted, I don't think I would have reached that conclusion and then I would have stayed there indefinitely. It makes me shudder now to think how that would have impacted the rest of my pregnancy and birth, and even my life today.

Looking back I now realise that by taking a conscious approach to my first pregnancy, I was not only able to avoid choosing major surgery for my first birth, but I was unknowingly creating a strong foundation of emotional resilience that would help to keep me from slipping into a subsequent bout of prenatal depression and the inevitable consequences that would likely follow.

Living Consciously

I touched on the idea of taking a conscious approach to pregnancy, but living consciously isn't limited to pregnancy and birth. It's something we can all do at any time, if we're ready and open to it.

Put simply, living consciously is being deliberate and mindful about your choices and conscious of their consequences. Many people live unconsciously from moment to moment and allow themselves to be carried by the current of life, instead of choosing to pick up an oar and paddle in a certain direction.

Bill Harris in his book *Thresholds of the Mind* describes being conscious like this: "Instead of being an automatic response mechanism, responding to the world based on unconscious rules, beliefs, fears, and limitations, he is able to consciously evaluate each situation, in the moment, and instantly and instinctively know exactly what to do and how to respond in order to gain the most resourceful outcome, both for himself and for others."

As with most things, to help you get your head around this perhaps it's easier to start with what the opposite of being conscious is; being UNconscious.

What is being UNconscious?

The personal growth expert and author Steve Pavlina describes people living unconsciously as those "whose conscious minds remain underdeveloped [and] often suffer from cluttered and unfocussed thinking. Needless worries, trivial distractions, inaccurate observations, false beliefs, and negative emotions run rampant through their thoughts, and most of the time they aren't even aware of it. It's like being stuck in a mental fog."

The personal growth expert Bill Harris says this on living unconsciously *"If you are unconscious, it appears that life is just happening, and, as a result you tend to feel like a victim, especially in situations where what happens is unpleasant."*. Victims tend to feel like they're not in control over what's happening to them. They also tend to look externally for support in "fixing" the situation they're in. This can make them quite passive. It's not hard to see how birth can play into this. Feeling like a victim can mean that they don't feel able to change their situation, because in their minds, the control or the solution lies elsewhere. And we all know how hard it is to change others! Much easier to change ourselves.

Living consciously is something that can begin at any point in your life, but the onset of becoming a parent is one of the best excuses to start. For one of my *Fear Free Childbirth* podcast episodes, I interviewed a mother, Laura, about her positive birthing experience. When I went back to edit the chat, I was struck by how conscious and deliberate Laura was in how she approached her pregnancy. Despite her first pregnancy not being planned, the minute Laura found out she was pregnant it really focussed her mind and was the trigger for setting in place the beginnings of a huge life shift. In the midst of a successful career, Laura began planning her exit strategy from corporate work so she could create a life that would enable her to be there for her children while still doing fulfilling work.

Listening to Laura, it's clear that she's a woman who is calm and measured, and who consciously and deliberately took the steps she needed to help her to prepare mentally and emotionally for her life as a mother and parent. This is what she says about pregnancy, which sounds to me a lot like a conscious pregnancy: "Pregnancy is the perfect opportunity to take the time to reflect and understand what kind of parent you want to be, what you want that relationship to look like with your child . . . to address what has brought you from your past to now, and how you want to move that forward positively."

I'm in complete agreement with her.

What Kind of Parent Do You Want to Be?

We can thank our parents for all the reasons that we're brilliant and all the reasons that we're not. They made us who we are through the way they are and the way they treated us as children (and still do). Many people "inherit" their parents' habits, and unfortunately this includes the less-than-desirable ones. Many parents' behavioural patterns inevitably recreate themselves in their children. But they don't have to. It is possible to stop these behavioural and emotional patterns from being passed on with some self-reflection and healing.

When we find out that we're about to become parents, it's a good time to think about the legacy you want to leave behind, and I don't just mean in a big, fanciful way. I mean in your children. They will be your greatest creations and your greatest legacy. Would you prefer them to be a version of you with all the crap you wrestle with daily? Do you want them to struggle with the things you have struggled with? Do you want them to make the mistakes you have made? Or would you prefer them to have a clear slate so they can create their own path?

There is no need to pass on your crap. But the only way to stop those patterns from repeating is for you to face them and find a way to stop doing them. As Laura says, pregnancy is the perfect time to reflect on who you are, why you are the way you are, and whether that's the person you want to be for your children. Taking the time to do this kind of work during your pregnancy will not only help you to prepare for a positive birthing experience, but will also help you to become the parent you want to be and that your children need you to be.

Earlier I mentioned that by choosing to live consciously during my first pregnancy, I was unknowingly creating a strong foundation of emotional resilience that helped me to withstand the pummelling of depression in my second pregnancy, but actually, that's not all. When I think back to becoming a new mum, I don't recall feeling completely overwhelmed by the experience as so many new mums are.

Now don't get me wrong. Yes, I suffered from lack of sleep and wondering what the hell needed to be done with this new little human being. But I didn't feel like I was drowning. I felt like it was something I could just deal with, and that with patience and calmness, I'd figure it out. Sure, there were many moments of "Oh shit! I can't cope!" but they were short-lived; they were moments, not days or weeks. My life as a new mother was pretty lonely; my mum had died several years back and I had no family or friends close by that I could turn to, so when I say that I felt I coped, it wasn't because I had an army of people around me to help me. It was just me and my partner, both struggling to keep our businesses going while juggling being new parents and shoehorning childcare into our working day. Life wasn't easy by any means. Back then I would have given anything NOT to have a business and to just be on maternity leave. But that wasn't the life we had chosen.

Becoming parents is a phase in life that many people struggle with. A faltering relationship will have all its cracks exposed, and even if you do have a strong relationship, the lack of sleep and additional stress can seriously rock your relationship boat. Many couples don't survive the first year of parenthood because the additional stress on the relationship that a child brings can be too overwhelming. What can help you through this is a strong foundation of emotional resilience and emotional awareness. The resilience will help you to withstand the inevitable extended periods of stress, while the awareness will help you to navigate this new terrain more easily. That's not to say that you won't experience challenges and testing times; it simply means that you're better equipped to deal with whatever comes your way.

I interviewed Elly Taylor, the author of *Becoming Us*, which is a book about becoming a family and how that affects your life and relationship as a couple. She says,

> *After "pregnancy and birth" and before "parenting," there's a very big and very important (but often overlooked) stage of parenthood, a time of adjustment to the changes every couple experiences when two becomes three. . . . A new baby, means a new mother, a new father, and a new family. . . . Change also brings opportunity for those who recognize it: invitations for insight, seeds for growth; windows for really knowing the fullness and truth of ourselves; and to learn valuable lessons in life and love.*

Elly highlights the important distinction between parenting (the act of being a parent and the relationship you have with your child) and parenthood (how your relationship as a couple changes to become parents as well as partners). In her book she talks at length about what you can both do during pregnancy to help you to prepare for parenthood. She believes that pregnancy is a great time to prepare, because you're able to do so without the pressure, distraction, and responsibility of another little human being.

So, if we feel compelled to bring more consciousness into our lives as a result of becoming parents, how might that look exactly? In the next chapter I explore how we might raise our consciousness during our pregnancy and how that might impact your birthing experience.

Chapter Four

Raising the Consciousness of Pregnancy and Birth

Conscious Communication
When I first became a mum, my sister-in-law passed me the book *The Baby Whisperer* by Tracy Hogg to help me to navigate this treacherous new terrain. As it happened, I didn't consult any other parenting books, as this book really resonated with me. It became my bible, and I was thrilled when I was able to get my daughter to sleep through the night by the middle of her second month. I am eternally grateful to Hogg's EASY* routine and her recommendation to swaddle babies. I followed her advice to the T and it worked for my baby. I'm not saying it will work for everyone, but it did for me and that's why I turned to it a second time for my second daughter.

EASY stands for Eat, Activity, Sleep, You time and is a three-to-four-hour cycle in which you move through these activities in this order in a regular and predictable way that provides security and routine to your baby.

There was one other important thing that I learned reading this book, and that was to talk to my daughter as if she could understand everything I was saying her. Tracy encourages you to walk your new baby around the home once you get home from hospital (if you went!) in order to introduce them to their new home. She also encourages you to talk to them constantly to let them know what you're doing and about to do - things like "I'm going to change your nappy / prepare the bath / put you to bed," etc. Essentially, you're treating your baby with respect and as if they're a person (which they are) rather than an object or an inferior being. This advice resonated with me and I always speak to my daughter, letting her know what's happening and what I'm thinking, planning, or doing. I'm sure this is why so many women talk to themselves - once you start, it's hard to stop! I'm a dab hand at this now. It felt pretty weird at the beginning, but these days you'll find me narrating my life even when I'm on my own.

This idea of treating children as little human beings in their own right, as a person with thoughts and feelings, isn't a new one. It was first put forward by the infamous French psychoanalyst Françoise Dolto. Dolto, whose work dominated most of the twentieth century, was well known for her work with babies and children. She wrote over thirty books as well as hosted a radio show, which made her a household name in France. Incredibly, she is hardly known in the English-speaking world, and yet she changed the face of French parenting, with her legacy still being felt today.

When Dolto was a young girl, she remembers thinking to herself, "When I'm older, I'll try to remember what it's like to be young," and that's what she did. The ideas that she introduced were extremely controversial in their day, and yet they make so much sense today that it seems almost strange that we didn't believe that at some point in time. The idea that is the most interesting for me is:

Your baby is a person and deserves the respect and attention that you would afford another human being

In terms of how this manifests itself in how we communicate with our child, Dolto suggested that we adopt her aptly named "Parler Vrai" style of communication. If I had to translate this, I'd say it's *speaking consciously* or *conversing mindfully*, which is about speaking *with* your baby as opposed *to* your baby. Dolto reminds us that we cannot lie to our subconscious and that the Truth is known deep down, whether that's within you or within your baby. For me, the important aspect here is *intention*. Your baby may not understand the words you're using, but he or she will definitely understand the intention behind those words, and intention is not something we can hide or misdirect. It forces us to be authentic and transparent with our children, but more importantly, it forces us to be authentic with ourselves. If we kid ourselves about who we are and why we're doing what we're doing, not only are we pursuing a path that is destined for unhappiness and unfulfillment, but we're also failing to create a strong foundational relationship with our children. A relationship that is built on trust and transparency has the potential to offer you one of the most fulfilling life experiences.

The thing is, it's not always easy to simply start being transparent and authentic. These are things that many people struggle with. Being authentic is something we work towards as we let go of being who we *think* we need to be and simply accept who we are, warts and all. This in itself can require you to face up to fears such as not being good enough or not being liked or accepted, or being rejected. This is all par for the course for those on the journey to consciousness and is not limited to pregnant mamas.

Positive Prenatal Enrichment

There are countless books and blogs advising expecting parents to happily embrace pregnancy and to shower their unborn baby with love and affection, that this is nothing new. For many parents-to-be it feels so completely natural and intuitive to welcome a new member of the family in such a way that it is rarely questioned. But there is quite a bit of research that's been carried out that shows how valuable it is for your unborn child to receive what is now known as *positive prenatal enrichment.*

The first study that measured the outcome of prenatal stimulation on babies and parents was carried out in California using the programme *Prenatal Classroom: A Parent's Guide for Teaching Your Baby in the Womb,* written with psychologist Marc Leher. The results were published in 1986 and they found **significant differences in early speech, physical growth, parent-infant bonding, and success in breastfeeding**[2]. The study was repeated in 1988 where similar trends were observed as well as **superior Apgar scores, high maternal ratings of the babies, and births that were "easier than expected."**[3]

This programme inspired an ambitious programme at the Huachiew Hospital in Bangkok, created by obstetrician Chairat Panthuraamphorn, which starts at twelve weeks gestation, where "test results show definite physical, mental, and emotional advantages to those in the stimulated groups (Panthuraamphorn, 1993). These babies showed significantly greater height and head circumference, fine and gross motor performance, and speech and language acquisition. They also smiled and laughed at birth - something rarely seen in the West."

And finally, a massive research project carried out in Caracas, Venezuela, which studied six hundred families randomised into experimental and control groups[4]. Extensive measurements were made at two days, one month, eighteen months, and three years of age. Led by psychologist Beatriz Manrique, the program aimed at complete and integrated bio-psycho-social development of children through adequate stimulation, training, and nutrition. Prenatal enrichment was accomplished in a thirteen-week course of two hours per week, using the guidebook *Answer Your Baby*, which teaches techniques of communication.

The results showed that the babies in Caracas demonstrated superior skills across the board (motor, visual, language, memory and auditory). Interestingly, the mothers also displayed increased levels of confidence, they were more active in labour and they enjoyed better breastfeeding rates as well as improved family bonding and cohesion.

These pieces of research make a strong case for connecting with and communicating to your baby as early as possible. In fact, you can start communicating to your baby long before conception. There are many conscious doulas I know who will help you to call and invite your baby into your lives and let it know that you are ready for them to make an appearance earthside.

As parents we strive to provide the best for our children - enrolling them in extracurricular activities, sending them to the best schools and universities - but perhaps we need to focus more on the time of their creation and growth. By nurturing our babies in utero and as babies, we can help them to grow into strong, capable, and intelligent beings who are more likely to thrive and succeed.

As pregnant mothers-to-be we start to make changes to our behaviours, stopping ones that are deemed damaging for our unborn child (such as drinking and smoking) and adopting new behaviours that are considered helpful (eating healthfully, exercising), but it appears that we shouldn't stop there. By taking time to connect and communicate to our unborn babies, we are developing a healthy habit of respect and relating to our babies that has far-reaching effects.

I know, it can seem that as a pregnant woman the list of things you need to start and stop doing is never-ending. It's all about the baby now, and it can feel like you and your needs disappear. And in some ways, that's how it is. Becoming a mother means having responsibility for another human being, and so your needs will fade into the background. That doesn't mean that it's a permanent thing, and it's always a question of balance - again, not an easy one to manage. I don't want to sit here and be the one to give you this huge, long list of things to do; instead I want to let you know that these are things that you *could* do and why you might want to do them. It's then up to you to decide consciously and mindfully whether you want to.

When I was pregnant, I decided that I wanted to do as much as I could to help my kids be healthy. As someone who was besieged with eczema, asthma, and allergies as a child, I wanted to do what I could to prevent my kids having those afflictions too. Even though I'm aware there are conditions and diseases that are much worse, when you have those issues as a child and you see other kids around you who don't have them, it can feel very isolating. I was picked on and bullied because of my eczema. I couldn't take part in all the exercises and games lessons because of my asthma and we couldn't have pets (still can't, in fact!) because of my allergies. Growing up, my confidence and self-esteem were affected because of how my skin looked, and even today my eczema holds me back in lots of silly ways that seem like nothing, but that have a great impact on my life. I wanted to do *everything* that I could to NOT pass that onto my children so they could be free of those kind of experiences. So, for me, living consciously during my pregnancy was important.

What Does a Conscious Pregnancy Look Like?

I want this book to help you as practically as possible, so I'd like to wrap up this little venture into living consciously by sharing with you the things you can do during your pregnancy to help raise your level of consciousness. However, as much as I like practical things, some of the things on this list are quite "big," and by that I mean that many of them are not the kind of things you can do over a weekend but instead require a more long-term approach. Having kids and parenting is a long-term game too, though, so I'm sure you'll get the gist.

These are in no particular order and there may be some overlap, but I hope that some of them help you to live more consciously.

Make careful, intelligent, and deliberate decisions

This means educating yourself about birth: exploring the various birthing options; understanding the potential questions you may be asked from healthcare professionals and thinking through your possible responses; understanding how the birth process affects the woman's body and how birth can be affected by the environment and interactions with others.

When you make a decision mindfully and from an informed perspective and without fear, you're much more likely to be able to live with your decision without regret or guilt. Guilt has a habit of eating you up inside for years to come and is best avoided.

Maintain a positive emotional state regardless of circumstance

This is not about positive thinking, or at least the shallow version of positive thinking that gets a bad rep everywhere. Many people mistake positive thinking for simply denying the crappy aspect and just focussing on the positive. I'm not suggesting that you deny the negative aspect to an experience. Instead, I'm suggesting you embrace the experience fully, recognising the negative that exists within it, but also looking for the positive. And then, crucially, retaining your focus on the positive and using that focus to help you through it.

Building a strong foundation of emotional resilience helps you with this because it means you will be better able to respond flexibly and positively to whatever situation may arise. Good or bad things don't happen to us; it's the interpretation we give those things that carries the meaning, and that's the bit we get to choose. Why choose to think of the thing you're experiencing as bad? Even if it is "bad" it won't last. The only thing we can be sure of in life is that everything changes. This means that if things are bad, they won't be for much longer. But equally, if things are good, appreciate them, because things will soon change!

In all good there is bad, and in all bad there is good. Everything is about balance, and too much of a good thing can become bad. Water is good for you, but drink too much and it will kill you. When you're in a strong emotional place, you're better able to identify the good in a situation so that you don't internalise it as bad. Gratitude is a wonderful place to escape to in times of need. In focussing on what we DO have, and not what we DON'T, we can find a way through difficult times.

When I lost my mother to cancer, I was thirty years old. It was six weeks from her diagnosis to her death, and it was the beginning of the darkest period of my life, which continued into the months that followed. While I was going through it, it was awful, but coming out the other end, I realised how lucky I was to go through what I had in the way that it unfolded. There was so much for me to be grateful about and I've always focussed on those aspects of that experience. Losing a parent is something we all have to go through and it will never be easy, but I chose to look for and focus on the positives. Now when I have crappy experiences, I choose to look for the positive when I'm in it, rather than waiting until afterwards. This helps me deal with what I'm facing and remain positive, even if I'm feeling rubbish and down. It is possible to feel crap AND be positive!

During your pregnancy, you might feel overwhelmed by the pregnancy symptoms you're experiencing, but perhaps there are positive aspects waiting to be discovered. I used to be super frustrated at my exhaustion and fragility, but once I accepted that I needed to slow down and simply do less, I grew to appreciate taking a slower approach to life and the things that we notice and become aware of as a result of slowing down. I used to speed about too much. I've retained some of this slowness now as I've grown to appreciate it. My various illnesses during pregnancy forced me to seek out natural alternatives, which have served me well since. I wouldn't have come across many of these things if I hadn't been forced to due to circumstance.

Develop empowering beliefs and purge the disempowering ones

Identify any beliefs that don't support a positive childbirth experience and address them. Then find ones that do and embrace them. This isn't just limited to your upcoming birth. Extend this to other aspects of your life.

When trying to strengthen a belief, seek out examples of it in action. So if you want to develop the belief that birth is natural and something you can do confidently, listening to other women share their positive birthing experiences will help you to do that. This is why I like to feature so many women sharing their positive birthing experiences on my *Fear Free Childbirth* podcast. Nothing beats listening to a woman talking about her birthing experience; hearing her voice and her conviction is powerful and does wonders for shifting your beliefs.

Understand your own thought processes, emotions, and behaviours

Dig deep to understand your own emotional landscape and address any things that might cause problems for you during birth or motherhood. This aspect can feel overwhelming, but making a deliberate attempt to address this is a great start. This is a journey, not a singular task, so as long as you take the first step, you're good to go. Then take another, and another.

This is a huge part of what this book is about. I don't believe we can isolate birth as an experience to prepare for because birth represents life. In preparing for birth, we're in effect preparing to fully live our lives and express who we truly are. There is no limit to this aspect of living consciously, only the limit you place on it.

Stay focussed on what's important and tune out distractions

During pregnancy (and in life), what's important is your family, your health, and your emotional well-being. What's less important is the type of pram you buy or the colour of the nursery. Consumer items and material things are distractions; what's real and what will affect you and your family's life day-to-day and in the future is your health, your relationships, how you feel, and how you deal with what happens to you.

Build an accurate model of reality

This is about understanding how things are and the possibilities that exist. When it comes to birth, many women focus on a narrow view of those possibilities, rather than the full spectrum. A lot of airtime, whether on TV or even during conversations among women, is given to birthing horror stories or when birth goes wrong. What we hear less about are those birth stories where the mother was enjoying it or wasn't in pain. These too are possibilities, yet we don't hear about them very often. In fact, we hear about them so seldom that many women don't think it's possible to give birth and not experience pain. This is simply not the case. That's not to say a pain-free birth is something we can all achieve, but it's a possibility, and a pretty good one.

Seeking examples of positive birth stories will help you to realise that having a positive birthing experience is a possibility, much more than "preparing" by watching medical dramas or reality TV shows. Some women mistakenly believe that watching shows like *One Born Every Minute* will help them to prepare for the reality of birth. What watching shows like that actually does is show you a narrow view of birth: the medical, hospitalised possibility. So, yes, on some level you're preparing, but you're really doing something far more damaging than that.

When you prime your subconscious for a particular possible outcome, you're increasing your chances of experiencing that outcome. Our mind needs a goal to focus on. We can either give it a goal consciously, or let it pick one at random based on what we've focussed our attention on. By choosing to watch dramatic versions of birth, we're in effect providing our mind with a goal, but it might not be the one we want. Be selective in how you prepare your mind for birth by ensuring that you have a good understanding of the possibilities that exist, and then focus your preparation and your attention on the outcome you want, not the one you want to avoid.

Regularly connect and communicate with your baby

Build a relationship with your baby early on in your pregnancy so that your baby is used to a two-way dialogue and trusts you. During birth there needs to be trust between the two of you. Trust that you're both capable and confident of doing what needs to be done and that you can rely on each other. Just as you need to have trust with your partner, trust with your baby is also important.

Letting your baby know that they are loved and wanted, and that a special place exists for them here in your life, is such a great way to let your baby know that they are welcome in this world. Invite your partner to communicate with your baby too. Communicate with your baby verbally or through thought and intention. Just use whatever feels easier for you. If it feels right, you might also want to thank them for choosing you to be their parent. Perhaps acknowledge their decision to come and join you in physical form, and let them know that you are grateful and ready for their arrival.

Make time for yourself

Your pregnancy is a good time to start penciling in some "me" time. If this is your first pregnancy, you probably haven't had to think of this before, the idea of *putting aside time for you*. But soon your time will be absorbed by so many other demands that "me" time will become scarce. Get your practice in while you can! Mothers often feel guilty for taking some "me" time, so by getting used to doing this in your pregnancy, you're preparing yourself for taking time out, which should help alleviate any potential guilt down the line.

Use this time to simply "be" and appreciate this transitional moment in your life. Take time to contemplate the significance of bringing a new life into this world and absorb the beauty and importance of what you are experiencing. You could take nature walks or do some meditating. This time that you spend alone will allow you the opportunity to process all the feelings of becoming a parent, facilitating the emergence of this new role.

Create space in your life for your baby

Many couples who are expecting their first baby do not intentionally create the space for a new person in their life, particularly if the baby wasn't entirely expected. It can be all too easy to try and bolt the baby onto your young, free, and independent life (I know because I was guilty of this!), but taking the time to think about what you need to let go of so that you can welcome your baby fully is worthwhile.

Take a closer look at any work, chores, hobbies, and relationships that are simply not compatible with family life. Be prepared to make changes to enable family life to flourish and thrive. Often, family friction comes from this resistance to let go of the life habits that suited a younger person with no responsibilities. By accepting your new role sooner, you can avoid much of this, and importantly, it gives a clear message to your new family member that they are welcomed, valued, and loved.

Journal your pregnancy experience

Write about your thoughts and emotions during pregnancy. Aside from the physical changes that accompany pregnancy, explore your ideas around how you want to parent, the relationship you hope to have, and the qualities you expect to foster in your child. Not only will this be interesting to read years from now to see how things panned out, but it will be a wonderful gift for your baby.

Our pregnancy journey impacts our babies in ways that we might find hard to grasp. Babies develop their senses very early on in utero and will pick up on a lot of your thoughts and experiences. The emotions that you experience will affect your baby in quite profound ways, one of the key reasons to address your emotional well-being during pregnancy.

I worked with a mother who brought me her daughter to work on. Her three-year-old was a fussy eater, but only at home - at nursery she ate well. I started by asking the mother about her pregnancy. She told me that it was fine apart from some morning sickness. When I probed deeper, asking about the kinds of thoughts she typically had during her pregnancy, she said that due to her morning sickness, she couldn't face eating anything. She told me that one of the most dominant thoughts during her pregnancy was "I can't eat; I can't face it. I'll be sick." Is it any surprise that when her daughter was in her presence she couldn't eat either? She had been primed before birth to be wary of food around her mother.

My own daughters illustrate this to me very clearly. My eldest daughter had to put up with me on my rollercoaster journey from fearful to fearless. During my first trimester I was full of fear, and one of the biggest ones was the fear of pain of childbirth. During my second trimester I cleared my fears, and by my third trimester I was pretty much fear-free. My eldest daughter, despite being very bold and active, can also be quite fearful, especially when it comes to pain. As I write this she is five years old and even the slightest scratch is a big deal. The site of blood worries her enormously and she cannot bear the thought of the pain of peeling off a bandage. Pain was my biggest fear, and my fear of injections and seeing my blood being taken for blood tests is clearly manifesting in her now.

My youngest, on the other hand, is a completely different kettle of fish. She has no fear whatsoever. She's been leaping off the top bunk bed since her first birthday and happily goes head-first down the big kids' slide at the park. She is constantly covered in scratches and bruises because she's always jumping off things and getting into scrapes. But she never cries and just isn't bothered by hurting herself or seeing the resulting scratches on her skin. One holiday when she was about twenty months old, we watched her fetch a ball in the rose bushes. In doing so she scratched her arm on a thorn. We heard her say "Ouch" and then watched her fetch a wipe to clean the blood off her arm before carrying on playing with the ball. There was no fuss and no drama. I can't help but think about how different my mental state was during my pregnancy with her, and the different thoughts that were going through my head in both my pregnancies, and how they seem to play out in observing my daughters' behaviour.

I wish my mother had kept a journal of her pregnancy, because I'm sure it would have helped me in sorting my own head out. It's very likely that much of the stuff that I've had to wrestle with in life was picked up and embedded while I was being carried by her, or during my birth. Understanding the reasons why I might be the way I am and the origins of some of my thoughts and feelings would have made the task of clearing out my headspace a lot easier.

Journalling doesn't need to be limited to the pregnancy journey; it can done for the birth too. Not necessarily by you, though! Although you could journal after the event if you like. A Conscious Birthing doula that I know, Lisa-Jane, often journals during a birth with a couple. She'll take photos and capture precious moments and then share the journal and the photos with the couple afterwards. This is such a precious gift. Our childbirth experience is such an important event in our lives that leaves deep imprints in our very being. As with our lives in utero, our birthing experience can hold the key to many aspects of ourselves that we seek to better understand. To be able to offer an account of this time in your baby's life to your child when they're older could be the best gift you could ever give them. If there's one thing we all wrestle with, it's trying to figure out who we are and why we are the way we are. People spend thousands on therapy and personal development to get these answers, answers that very often lie within our in utero and childbirth experiences.

Detox from chemicals

Pregnancy often forces you to start seeking more natural alternatives due to the fact that if you're ill, you can't take antibiotics or many other medications. It was during my first pregnancy that I learned how I could maintain my health in a more natural way. My health cabinet at home now contains things like baking soda, aqueous iodine, colloidal silver, magnesium chloride flakes, essential oils, hydrogen peroxide, coconut oil, and apple cider vinegar. I've managed to keep most bugs at bay by turning to these, which has limited the family's use of antibiotics, which as we know are losing efficacy and abolish so much more in the body that simply the bad thing they're used to get rid of.

But this detoxing has now extended to chemicals that are used around the house. Cleaners, toothpastes, fragrances, etc., have also been replaced by kinder products that are less damaging to our bodies and also less damaging to the environment. As a mother, I've become more mindful of environmental concerns (and I was before, so now I'm even more so!). Our planet is our children's home, and they are the ones that will have to deal with the mess that our generation and the ones before us have created.

Discard your chemical cleaners and start cleaning your home with microfibre cloths and water, adding things like baking soda, castile soap, or vinegar. Remove the chemicals that you can from your home, laundry, kitchen, bathroom, and environment. It's no accident that pregnant mothers become extra sensitive to smells - don't ignore your senses! They're flagging things for a reason.

Work on your relationship with your partner

The greatest gift you can offer your future child is a loving relationship between his or her parents. If there are any unresolved issues between you and your partner, make a point to work on them before your baby arrives so you can welcome your child into a peaceful home. Devote time to your relationship, whether through therapy or counselling, simple open communication, or even a baby-moon. A happy couple and a happy home massively increases your chances of having a happy child.

The premise of this book is ultimately about clearing away all your head trash - the negative thoughts, feelings, and emotions - that stand between you and a stress-free pregnancy and a fear-free birth. But our head trash is more far-reaching than that. It's actually responsible for preventing you from connecting to who you really are. In choosing to live consciously, you are taking a deliberate decision to raising your consciousness. This is a very exciting and liberating journey to be on, although it's not always easy.

In doing the work required in letting go of our crap, we rediscover and reconnect with ourselves; we're in effect getting closer to expressing our true self, our essence, our Truth. Whichever way you prefer to articulate that idea, it represents the very core of who we are, and if when you have children you still are far from knowing or understanding that person, then being a parent will surely bring you closer.

What Does a Conscious Birth Look Like?

For me, there is a change that takes place from a conscious pregnancy to a conscious birth. During our pregnancy we find ourselves making active choices about all aspects of our life as we strive to raise our consciousness, from choosing to avoid chemicals to choosing new ways of thinking and behaving. But an important part of being conscious is also stepping out of our mind and *doing*, and making the shift into *being*. There is no event or activity that is more deserving of this state of being than birth. By the time birth comes around, it's time for the mind to step aside and let the body take centre stage. Being present will help to support you in supporting your body in this way.

A conscious birth is achieved by letting go and surrendering to the process, but this is not necessarily an easy thing to do if you have fears, anxieties, and distractions keeping your conscious mind busy. The value in using your pregnancy to prepare for birth cannot be denied. For some women, a conscious birth is when they are able to hand over their body and their mind is clear of thought and emotion. For them, the conscious part is all the preparation that they have undertaken that enables them to be that way during birth: choosing their birthing team, making emotional and mental preparations, and considering the choices around their birth.

A conscious birth can also be one in which the woman is totally present and aware of her body and her baby. She is able to notice what her thoughts are doing and she knows how to control them if she needs to. She is aware of her breath and her body and can make the changes she needs for support. A woman who consciously births like this can't be said to be in control, because control is an illusion that tricks us. Instead she is able to respond flexibly and calmly to what she becomes aware of in her mind, her body, and her baby.

You can't just rock up to a conscious birth on the day, not unless you've prepared for it, but that is what I hope to be able to help you with. By addressing the fears and the anxieties in your mind, you'll be much better placed to remain present. You'll also find it much easier to tune in to your body and your baby and respond accordingly. The journey to a conscious birth starts with raising your consciousness during pregnancy.

Chapter Five

Stress and Pregnancy

S tress is something we're all familiar with. Unfortunately, when
we're pregnant, being stressed can have some unpleasant side
effects, for both you and your baby. But it's not only stress we need to
worry about; depression and anxiety are worrying too. Dr Chamberlain cites that at least thirty studies since the 1950s have focussed on
the link between the emotional and mental state of the mother and
complications at birth and or abnormalities in the children[5].

From this extensive body of research into prenatal and perennial
psychology, Chamberlain (and Mikhael Aivanhov, 1982) has no doubt
of the extent to which education is constantly taking place between
mothers and their babies before birth, and how maternal well-being
affects the unborn baby.

In a study of over a thousand mothers tested for different degrees
of depression during pregnancy, researchers found depressed mothers
gave birth to babies who tended to be inconsolable and cry excessively
in correlation with their mother's depression scores[6]. Similarly, mothers
who are very anxious may give birth to babies who are cranky, colicky,
cry excessively, and have difficulties feeding[7].

Feeling unhappy during pregnancy can sometimes have significant
consequences. When researchers studied the medical records of a

group of severely disturbed children and adolescents, they found the majority had been born to unmarried mothers who had not planned the pregnancy, to mothers who felt unhappy about being pregnant, to mothers who lived in family discord, to mothers who felt emotionally rejected for being pregnant, or to mothers with more physical health problems[8]. Chamberlain goes on to suggest that "chronic stress during pregnancy may very well affect the later well-being of the children."

In talking about mental states such as stress, anxiety, and depression, I think it's important to make the point that even though as pregnant women we must strive to minimise our levels of stress as much as possible, it doesn't mean that we should avoid feeling any sort of negative emotion whatsoever. Life is full of highs and lows, and during the nine months of a pregnancy many things can happen, from moving house or losing a job to a family death. If something like this were to happen to you during your pregnancy, there is no need to start feeling guilty for the sake of your child. Experiencing the normal range of human emotions is fine, and if that includes grief, loss, rejection, or sadness then it's important that you accept those emotions and process them. Your baby is learning how to be a human being by the example you set, and that means learning how to handle negative emotions too. Where things start to have a negative impact on your body and your baby is when the emotion is chronic and never-ending.

One known link between stress and your baby is this: maternal stress increases your baby's chance of having eczema. This one is pretty close to my heart as I've had really bad eczema most of my life since being a tiny tot. So when I came across this research, from the National Center for Child Health and Development, Allergy Division in Tokyo[9], it made a lot of sense. After analysing data from 896 pairs of mothers and children (474 boys and 422 girls), this is what they found:

- 47% of atopic eczema in babies occurs due to stress during pregnancy
- Maternal anxiety during pregnancy is a risk factor for the onset of infantile atopic eczema at six to eight months of age

When my mother was pregnant with me, she hid her pregnancy because she was worried that her employer would find out and fire her (it was the seventies!). She was supporting my dad while he was doing his PhD, so her income was critical. This was an important motivating factor for me in trying to achieve a stress-free pregnancy because I'm all too familiar with how horrid eczema can be, especially growing up. If there was anything I could do to help my own child avoid having to experience any one of those, then I wanted to try. Whether we're pregnant or not, there is always a benefit to be had from strengthening our emotional resilience, and for most people this starts with actively de-stressing. Stress is the beginning of the slippery slope to anxiety and depression, so if we can start by tackling stress, then we're more likely to be able to avoid its uglier sidekicks: anxiety and depression.

The Primary Causes of Stress

I n order for us to think about eliminating stress, it can be useful to understand a little bit more about where it comes from, or at least what causes it. Essentially, stress is caused by the following (*once you see this list, you'll understand why pregnancy and childbirth can be so damn stressful!*):

- Fear
- Physical exertion
- Medical illness
- Adverse reactions to medication
- Environment

Let's take a closer look at these and how they affect and are affected by pregnancy and childbirth.

Medical condition or illness

When you're affected by a medical condition or illness, it puts physical stress on the body. As our body is an interconnected system, when one thing is out of kilter, other parts of the system are affected too. On top of that, your body is spending its energy trying to heal you, so there is additional demand on your body. The body would find all this quite stressful, but when you're pregnant, your body has already got its plate full MAKING A BABY so things could easily go off the chart for you. Things are not helped by the fact that you probably won't be able to take any medication for whatever is affecting you, simply because you're pregnant. But there is an added dimension here: how you *feel* about what is happening to you. In addition to physical stress, you may also be experiencing *emotional stress*.

Let's say you've got really bad heartburn. How are you likely to feel about that? Possible responses might include:

Response #1

"Oh, this heartburn is annoying... all part of pregnancy, though... I'd better take some ginger / cut back on spicy fatty foods, etc."
Nature of response: Mainly internal thoughts.

Response #2

"Oh, no! Not heartburn again! It's so uncomfortable. I can't wait for this to end."
Nature of response: Mainly internal thoughts, but some verbal comments too.

Response #3

"I hate this bloody heartburn! It's so frustrating! I can't sleep! It hurts! I wish it would stop! Grrrrr!"
Nature of response: Internal thoughts with a lot of verbal expression of thoughts. Frequent complaining to those around you that might include gesticulation with arms, or the raising of voice in frustration.

Which one do you think would be typical of you? Be honest!

You'll notice that response three is a much more stressed response than response one. Response one is from someone who appears to be taking the heartburn in stride and accepts that it's part of her pregnancy. Response two, while still fairly accepting of her condition, shows a slightly shorter fuse with it; however, she still appears to be coping with it. Contrast this with response three, which shows somebody who is noticeably stressed by her condition. Her stress might be because this is how she responds to most things, or it might be because she's been experiencing this for four months now and it's REALLY DOING HER HEAD IN! Maybe she started at response one, but the continuation of the heartburn, along with all her other symptoms, is starting to wear her down. Whatever the reason for her response, if response three is now her modus operandi, then her body will also be experiencing the stress response, which will exacerbate the heartburn (thus creating a never-ending loop!).

So in this situation, if you could respond differently emotionally to your physical symptoms, then you could influence how much stress your body will experience. Fortunately, this is something you can do. At its simplest, you can just decide not to get annoyed by such things and accept that all this is part of pregnancy. In saying that, I realise it sounds easier said than done, so luckily it's possible to address your emotional response and tone it down, if not neutralise it entirely. Continue reading to find out how, but for now I want you to be aware that HOW you respond to something is often more stressful than the thing you're experiencing.

Physical exertion

The very physical nature of pregnancy and childbirth means that this is clearly one of the main causes of stress. Of course, the extent to which this affects you will be down to your general state of health and well-being. If you're fit and in good shape, and you exercised regularly before you became pregnant, then you will more than likely find it easier to cope with both your pregnancy and childbirth. However, if you're not in the best of shape, this physical stress could be quite significant for you.

Now, as above, there is the additional element to consider: the emotional stress. How you feel about the physical demands of pregnancy will affect your stress response too. Are you *resisting* what is happening to you? You know, denying it? Trying to carry on as normal? Or are you accepting it and slowing down?

This was one of my main stressors in the early part of my second pregnancy. I thought I could carry on as normal - like I did in my first pregnancy - but my body had other plans. I would get so frustrated at not being able to function in the same way, and at being so tired and hungry all the time. Once I totally let go of "how things were" and "how I wanted things to be" and accepted that my body needed all this energy to create a little person, I found it much easier to cope. It involved having to let go of things I wanted to do. I had to put my business on hold, my normal household chores and organisation pretty much stopped, and I couldn't play with my daughter in the same way; in short, I had to stop doing lots of things that were very important to me. It was super hard, but once I *accepted* that this was how life needed to be, it became much easier. And it was a relief! It reminded me to get back to living in the present (which I had clearly forgotten), and that this was just a transient phase. My unborn daughter needed this from me.

Adverse reactions to medication

This one is highly unlikely to affect you during your pregnancy as most medication is off limits, but it can certainly start wreaking havoc with things during childbirth if you've chosen to accept being induced or given pain relief. What makes this additionally stressful is that it's so hard to predict. There can be no way of knowing if we're about to take a medication that will trigger nasty side effects, some of which can be worse than the thing it's trying to help us with.

This aversion to medicine during pregnancy might seem like a real chore on the surface, but it can have a positive consequence. Whenever things came up for me that would normally be helped by medicine, I would seek a natural alternative to heal my body. During both of my pregnancies, I learned a lot about the natural approach to healing. I was regularly surprised at the speed at which I healed from various ailments during my pregnancies, including things for which I would have normally been prescribed antibiotics. It was an eye-opener for me, and something that has stayed with me post-pregnancy.

Environment

Your environment can be quite significant stress-wise during both your pregnancy and your childbirth, but it's during labour and birth that it can have the most impact. It's really important that your environment is as calming and as relaxing as possible on D-Day, so try to plan in advance to help reduce the likelihood of your environment causing you stress on the Big Day.

If you're choosing to have a hospital birth, think about what you can bring with you to make the environment nicer. Soft lighting, photos, pillows and cushions, music, aromatherapy? Find out what the hospital will accept. Maybe visit the rooms in advance so that you can get a sense of how it will be, rather than get a pleasant surprise, or nasty shock, on the day!

Fear

This one is a biggie! This is why I kept it until last. This whole book is about fear so I'll keep it short and sweet. To be honest, in the context of this book, when we talk about fear, we could just as well as be talking about *anxiety*. And you may be asking yourself what the difference is between the two, so let's just take a quick look.

Fear vs. Anxiety - What's the difference?

Fear and anxiety produce similar physical responses to certain dangers: muscle tension, sweaty palms, increased heart rate, and shortness of breath are just a few of the physiological symptoms you might experience. These bodily reactions are part of the fight-or-flight stress response that is hardwired into us for our survival (at least it was important for our survival when we lived in caves, less so now; today we just need a Wi-Fi connection and chargers).

Many experts would have you believe that there are important differences between the two, and while we might not agree, I think it's pretty useful for us to have a peek, as the distinction is quite useful for us in the context of childbirth. According to authors Kaplan and Sadock, anxiety is "a diffuse, unpleasant, vague sense of apprehension " and is often a response to an imagined, imprecise, or unknown threat. For example, let's say you're walking down a dark street. You might feel a bit apprehensive and have butterflies in your stomach, or be overcome with a sense of dread. These feelings are caused by the anxiety that is related to the *possibility* that a nasty stranger may jump out from behind a van and ask for your wallet, or worse. This anxiety is not the result of a *known* or *specific* threat because you don't know for sure that there's a nasty man lurking about. Instead, it's all in your head; you're *imagining* that there *might* be a nasty man. You may argue with that, saying, "Well, I'm in a dodgy part of town that's littered with questionable characters on every street corner, so I'm pretty confident that this is a real threat," but it only becomes real when a man actually appears.

Then fear kicks in.

Fear is an emotional response to a *known* or *definite* threat. Staying in our darkened street, let's say someone does appear from behind that rusty old van and holds a knife up in your face, asking for your mobile phone and wallet; this would trigger your fear response. In this case, the danger is real, definite, and immediate. While the physiological sensations you experience in both these scenarios might be similar, your *fear* response would be probably be significantly more intense than your *anxiety* response.

We can see from this example that there is a difference, but it's pretty subtle, because if you *believe* that the danger is real, as opposed to *imagined,* then your body will react accordingly.

When it comes to childbirth, many women may cite a fear of pain, or a fear of complications, whereas in reality these are anxieties, because until the pain is there, or until the complication has been confirmed by the doctor, it's just imagined. But if you *believe* that these things are certainties, and "that's just how childbirth is" then your body will not be able to tell the difference and will trigger the fear response - the stronger one of the two. Unfortunately, when it comes to pain, a strong fear response is the last thing you want (I'll explain this fully later on).

So, is it just a question of vocabulary or linguistics? It may well be. Think about how you describe your thoughts, feelings, and sensations in your head. Often, just changing the language we use to describe something can elicit a very different response in our bodies, which can therefore impact our actual experience.

Imagine you're about to go on a roller coaster, a super swirly one that goes upside down with lots of steep twists and turns. As you sit in your seat waiting for it to go up the first steep slope before the big drop that starts the ride, how are you feeling? Excited? Scared? A bit of both? When you think about it, your physical response is quite similar, whether you're excited or scared: butterflies in your stomach, sweaty palms, racing heartbeat.

Now imagine you have to give a talk in front of a load of people. How does that make you feel physically? Do you get butterflies in your tummy? Sweaty palms? Racing heartbeat? And this time, how would you describe that feeling to yourself? Nervous? Excited? Scared? Terrified? In this situation, the words that you use in your mind to label the physical feeling will loop back into your feelings.

So if you choose to describe the butterflies in your tummy and your sweaty palms as fear (scared, terrified), then your mind will start to seek out rational reasons why you're right to feel fear: you might stammer or get your words wrong and look stupid. As your mind busies itself worrying about stammering or getting your words wrong, guess what? You get your words wrong! You accomplish what you focussed on. Now, what if you described those same bodily sensations as *nervous* and *excited* instead? In your head you tell yourself that being nervous is perfectly reasonable, and that it will soon pass. In this instance, your mind isn't worrying about messing up your words, which means you probably won't.

Your mind never wants you to be wrong, so it will always seek and find evidence to support what you believe to be true. Hence the power of beliefs. Change your beliefs and your mind will seek, and find, evidence to support those instead.

Physical feeling ➡ **Labelled by the mind** ➡ **Affects physical feeling**

Think about how that might work with pain. But more on that later.

Fear (perception of danger) is quite a broad term, and we can experience it to varying degrees. For example, if we've got a mild or small amount of fear, we might experience that as nervousness, concern, or apprehension. Mild to moderate fear might be experienced as agitation, anxiety, and worry. And moderate to extreme fear might be experienced as feeling frightened, scared, terrified, or hysterical.

So remember this:

- Fear ALWAYS produces an associated response of stress (fight-or-flight).
- The degree of stress response is DIRECTLY proportional to the degree of fear: the greater the fear, the more intense the stress response.

A stress response in the body will be triggered EVERY time we perceive we are in danger (experience fear) with each fear message producing an associated stress response. Now, even though we might not feel the effects of a stress response reaction, one is still happening. There's no "Get Out of Jail" card here. We can't escape it. We will experience the stress response no matter where we sit on the fear-o-meter. Lots of people assume that we only experience the stress response with the stronger forms of fear, such as feeling frightened, terrified, or scared, but actually, we experience it with fear at ANY level. Even if you're merely nervous, concerned, or worried, your body is under stress.

It's important to realise this, particularly in relation to childbirth, because the stress response in the body is public enemy number one for women in labour.

What Are Your Stress Triggers?

If you're going to have a stress-free pregnancy, our first step is to **iden-tify** those things that are causing you stress.

As I mentioned earlier, stress is caused by fear. Pregnancy is a huge time of change - in your life and in your body - so it's understandable that we feel fearful. We're fearful of the unknown. Fearful of what might go wrong. Fearful of the horror stories we've heard. There's a lot at stake, and if we believe everything we read or are exposed to concerning pregnancy and birth, there's a lot to be scared about. We simply don't know how our pregnancy is going to pan out. *Will I develop complications? How will I feel about my body changing? Will my hormones go crazy and give me nasties like gestational diabetes? What if my blood pressure goes off the chart? What if I develop a bad case of sciatica? How long is this morning sickness going to last? Am I going to feel this exhausted until I give birth?*

The stress response in the body can be triggered by low-level worry and distant concerns, as well as things you might quite clearly recog-nise as stressors in your life. Clue: if you find yourself saying "God, this is really stressing me out!!" obviously that particular thing is on your Stress List. What I want to help you with is identifying those things that contribute to that low-level hum of stress that's constantly there, so much so that you probably hardly notice it. But you're body is being affected by it, and so will Baby.

Now, the surprising thing here is that it's not as easy as it sounds. Why? Well, because many of the things that contribute to your stress are bubbling away under your radar. You've become so used to them, you probably don't realise how much they're adding to your overall feeling of stress. It's a bit like the electrical appliances in your house. In my lounge the TV, the cable box and the sound system all give off a low-level hum or frequency. When I sit in my lounge reading a book, I might well think it sounds quiet, but all these gadgets are actually making a noise, albeit a really tiny amount of noise. It's only when I go around to each one and actually switch the power off that the lounge becomes truly quiet. And it's only then that I realise how noisy they all were. I had just become so used to it that I hadn't noticed.

Well, that's what life stress is like too. You're being affected by lots of things in a low-level kind of way, but together they're all adding up to an overall feeling of stress. The problem with this is that because you're already in a stressed state (fairly mild probably), it doesn't take much to tip you over into a noticeable or visibly stressed state. But once you get rid of these everyday stress triggers, you'll look back and realise just how stressed you were. The added concern for pregnant women is that the body will experience the stress response as a result of these low-level stresses, and that means Baby will too. So these are super important to tackle.

Now, let's get one thing straight. When I say "get rid of the stress triggers," what I'm NOT saying is turn your life upside down and get rid of all the stressy people and things in it. Getting rid of or changing things like your house, your job, your car, your kids, and/or your partner would be a pretty hardcore solution to getting rid of your stress triggers. What I AM saying is change YOU, so that you stop *reacting* to those triggers. This way those things can still happen and those people can still behave that way, but now they just don't stress you out anymore. Changing *how we respond* to life changes our experience of life, so that's what I want to help you with.

Think about losing a job. Losing your job or being made redundant sucks, whichever way you look at it. Suddenly your regular source of income is threatened and you're going to need to find another job or source of income. Some people will find the news of being laid off super stressful and they'll panic. A ton of worries and fears will pile in: *What if I can't get another job? My life is going to change - am I going to like the new version? How am I going to be able to cope? etc.* Whereas for others, once they get over the initial stressy shock of it, they get excited or inspired to make a bigger change in their life. It might even be a relief if they didn't like their job anyway. Or they might see it as a chance to try something new and meet new people. They might still worry about income, but they're responding differently and this enables them to take on a different, more helpful perspective that is actually going to help them resolve the situation. This is what I mean when I talk about changing how you respond to something. You can't insure yourself against rubbish things happening to you, but you can choose to not allow them to affect you in the same way. Making that choice isn't always easy, as our default response is often hardwired into us. I want to help you to change this hardwired response, and it's not as hard as you think. But first we need to start by identifying the things that are contributing to your pregnancy stress levels.

To help you to start clearing your pregnancy stress, I've got two very simple questions that I want you to think about:

1. **What situations stress me out?** . . . or finish this sentence "*Situations or things that happen to me and stress me out include . . .* "
2. **What behaviour in others stresses me out?** . . . or finish this sentence "*People cause me stress when they . . .* "

Stressful Situations

This is going to include all sorts of situations, from the big-deal, life-changing ones like losing your job or breaking up with a partner, to the tiny life annoyances like missing your train or bus, or getting a parking ticket. But obviously, you need to come up with a list of situations that cause YOU stress*, not situations that you imagine are stressful to others. Some pregnancy things that might make it on your list is the constant need to pee, not being able to buckle or tie your shoes (can't reach!), having to find large parking places (so that you can easily get out of your car), or getting some unpleasant or unexpected test results from the midwife.

*Remember, when I talk of "stress," there is a varying scale of response that I'm referring to. To ensure that we clear the low-level hum I was referring to earlier, we have to include the stressful stuff that is at the lower end too, like discomfort, slight annoyances and being bugged by someone/something. But also there are the mildly stressful responses like frustration, strong dislike, exasperation and worrying. And at the top end, the super-stressful responses like strong fear, anxiety and panic. It'll probably be much easier for you to identify those things that trigger a super stressful response as these are more noticeable. It's the ones at the gentle end that might be harder, for the reasons I gave earlier; you've just become used to experiencing them so much that you don't really notice it.

Stressful Behaviour

This is going to include things that people say or do that cause you stress. It's surprising how many people start to treat you differently when you're pregnant. Some people have only the best intentions and want to help and look after you, but even their best intentions can wind us up the wrong way. Behaviours might include people touching your belly or constantly commenting on your body/shape/size, people not letting you have a seat on public transportation, or dealing with a patronising or unsupportive midwife or doctor.

Birth Prep Work

Take a pause for a moment to list the Situations and Behaviours that cause you stress. I'm sure reading this has already triggered a few things in your mind, so you may as jot them down while you're thinking about it.

How to Tell if You're Stressed by Something

You might think that you're pretty clear on what stresses you out and you'd be right. You are, on some level. You might be totally aware of what stresses you out, but sometimes you'll only figure it out with hindsight. How come? Well, because once whatever it is that's stressing us is no longer in our lives, we realise what a toll it was having on us. We only notice it once it's gone. Well, that's not helpful to us, especially if we're trying to stop it from affecting us. What if the thing never goes away, always rearing its ugly head? As D-Day approaches, it's even more important to get this stuff out of your life. So rather than just leave this thing floating around in your subconscious, I want to help you to raise your own awareness about your life stressors. It can be useful to think about *energy* when we talk about stress (or any negative emotional state), particularly *excess emotional energy*.

Have you got a friend who hates nothing more than other people being late? Yes? Are you thinking of someone? OK, now imagine this: You've arranged to meet your friend, let's call her Jane, for coffee, along with a couple of other friends. You arrive on time to find Jane already sitting comfortably in the cafe with her drink. You settle down and decide to wait for your other friends to turn up before ordering your drink. Five minutes passes and Jane starts getting fidgety; she's checking her watch, looking around to see if the others are arriving. Another five minutes passes and the fidgeting intensifies. But now there are strong sighs too. You ask her if everything is all right and she exclaims (in a slightly raised voice), "Well, Rachel and Sarah are late!" and as she says it, her hands start gesticulating as with particular emphasis on the word LATE. Another five minutes pass and she starts ranting about how she hates people being late and as she does, her arms are animatedly helping her to make her point. It's not pretty. Does that scene seem familiar to you?

Compare that to the time you were out with another friend of yours, Kate, who isn't bothered about other people being late. She would be quite happy to chat away with you while waiting for your other friends. She might check her watch occasionally, probably out of habit, but it wouldn't distract her from the chat she'd be having with you. If after ten minutes your other friends still haven't tuned up, she might mention that she hopes they're OK and that nothing's happened to them. Essentially the lateness of your friends is a non-event for her. It doesn't even cause a ripple. What concerns her more is their well-being. She is *neutral* when it comes to *lateness*; she can take it or leave it.

What's the main difference between these two scenarios? (Other than the fact that you'd probably much prefer being stuck in that cafe with Kate than with Jane.) The difference is *energy*. Jane's discontent with lateness brings up a lot of negative energy in her that needs to come out. It starts seeping out in her fidgety gestures, and as long as the trigger remains, the energy needing to be expressed increases. So there are deep, loud sighs that accompany the now more pronounced checking-of-watch and looking-around-to-see-who's-arriving gestures. As time goes on and the trigger causing the negative energy is still in place, things need to be cranked up a level to allow this energy to be expressed. This excess energy now starts to pour into the voice. The raised voice is then accompanied by even more intense hand gesticulation.

Now, some people might have a slightly different style. Rather than let the negative emotional energy seep out in a gradual, even fashion, as Jane did, they might try to keep it all suppressed. But this isn't going to last long. At some point it will need to come out, whether it's on that day or much later. And when it does, it'll be quite an explosion. In the meantime, the stress the mind and body will experience as they try to stifle this negative energy will be very damaging. Negative energy is always better out than in. You wouldn't dream of stopping a fart from coming out! (Unless you're in a lift!) Just the very idea of a toxic fart (it's waste matter, after all) being reabsorbed by the body is enough to make you realise that it's better out than in. It can be useful to think of negative emotional energy in the same way. The longer it stays in your body, the more toxic its effect on your mind-body system.

Without this excess negative emotional energy that needs to be released, we wouldn't see these types of reactions. And ultimately, what I want to help you to do with this book is to *neutralise negative emotional energy*. Energy that, if it were being retained in your mind and body, would be quite disruptive and damaging physically. But not only that, it would probably be pain-inducing on your D-Day.

In order for us to be able to neutralise this negative emotional energy, we first need to identify what's triggering its expression. To help you to do that, here is a list of the kind of responses that I'm referring to:

- Hand gesticulation: waving of hands; finger-pointing to emphasise certain words or phrases
- Changes in breathing: loud, vocal sighs; sharp intake of breath (stress response); shallow breathing (another sign of stress)
- Change in the voice: raised voice; faster delivery of words and phrases; maybe even tripping over some words
- Tension in the face and body: frowning; clenched jaw; tight shoulders; clenched fists
- Posture: leaning forward; rigid.

As you look at this list, you'll notice that each of these requires *energy*. The waving of your hands, the raised voice, the increased heart rate are the result of energy being expelled from deep within you, and based on what we're seeing, we can presume that it's negative energy, because these are rarely the signs of a super happy person.

This negative energy resides within you and its very presence already affects you in ways you may not realise. It might be contributing to some physical symptoms or conditions that you are afflicted by. When you come across a situation or a person that acts as a trigger, they are merely bringing something that is normally hidden to the surface. They are not *creating* that in you, and they are not the *cause*; they are merely the *trigger*, triggering something within you that needs to be expressed, addressed, and healed. For that, you can choose to be grateful, because without these triggers, you wouldn't know what you needed to work on. They are bringing you a gift.

This is a great attitude to adopt when faced with annoying situations and people. Life is merely presenting you with yet another thing that you need to work on in yourself. The world is simply a reflection of yourself. Once you neutralise the negative emotional energy that's triggered as a result of a particular situation or interaction with someone, then it's unlikely that you will be affected in the same way by that type of situation again. So don't get mad, just add it to your list and say "thank you."

Birth Prep Work

It's time for some more prep work. Find the list that you started in earlier and let's add to it. Think about the following questions and write anything down that comes to mind.

- *What happens in your life that triggers the need to express a load of negative energy?*
- *What do people say or do that triggers a response?*
- *What situations trigger a stress response for you?*

Chapter Six

Due Date Stress

I n the final month of pregnancy, your due date has the potential to be one of the main triggers of pregnancy stress, yet much of this stress can be avoided. To put it another way, there are things we can do early in our pregnancy to minimise this stress quite significantly, if not eliminate it entirely.

Stress is the LAST thing you want in the lead-up to the birth, because stress is the enemy of labour; the more stress you experience, the more likely you are to delay the arrival and/or the smooth progression of labour. This in itself compounds stress levels even more and can lead to all sorts of unwanted outcomes when it comes to the birth. So, if anything, you need to be completely stress-free at this point, not entering into a super stressful phase. What exactly is likely to cause you stress around your due date? I'm afraid a big part of it is people. There are two groups of people you need to be wary of, and believe it or not, your (well-meaning) friends and family are at the top of the list! The other lot includes the doctors, midwives, and obstetric consultants.

Your friends and family

Ask any mum and she will be more than happy to share with you the nightmare of THAT FINAL MONTH. Most conversations begin with the other person asking, "Is baby there yet?" or you nipping things in the bud by saying, "No! There's no baby yet!" or some other variation. This silliness usually starts a week or so BEFORE your due date, as people inevitably forget the date and/or wonder if Baby might have arrived early. These well-meaning friends appear to be under the illusion that if you had the baby, you decided to keep it completely to yourself and not mention it AT ALL to ANYONE WHATSOEVER, as new parents often do (NOT!).

What's more, keeping in line with many other pregnancy experiences, the world and their wife seem to think it's completely acceptable to comment on your body size, and what you should and shouldn't be doing to kick off the proceedings.

"Ooh, you're SOOOO BIG, it can't be long now!" - *Yeah, thanks for that! That makes me feel so much better!*

"Why don't you put your feet up and take it easy?" - *Because I have a life and putting your feet up for weeks is BORING!*

If baby insists on staying put, then it's not long before you start getting bombarded by a barrage of well-meaning yet unrequested advice. If you've only had this for a week, that might be OK, but after three weeks, it might really begin to wear you down. Especially when this well-meaning banter starts to crank up a level:

"Have you and [source of sperm] thought about having sex? You know . . . to bring the baby on?"

"Go and treat yourself to a curry!"

"Eating pineapple is meant to help - why don't you try that?"

"Have you tried stimulating your nipples?"

"You're bound to drop soon, you look MASSIVE!"

Do they honestly think that I don't know any of this? That I haven't spent most of my waking nights in between my frequent trips to the loo Googling "how to bring labour on" . . . I'm a full-fledged expert on things-that-trigger-labour AND I'M DOING ALL OF IT!!!!

The doctors, midwives, and obstetric consultants

As your due date approaches, if she hasn't already, your midwife will begin to ask you about what steps you would like to take, if and when you go past your due date. Would you like a sweep? How about an induction? Obviously, any discussions you have with your midwife will be dependent on the type of pregnancy you've had, the state of your health, and any signs from your baby. But if, on the whole, things have gone well for you and there is no medical reason for you to consider having anything other than a normal* birth, then the midwife will want to understand how you would like things to play out if baby doesn't arrive by a certain time (this is likely to be a week or so after your due date).

*I say "normal" knowing this means NOTHING, so what I really mean is . . . the birth you would like, whether that's a natural birth or water birth, a hospital birth or home birth.

Women's experiences with their healthcare providers vary wildly at this stage. On the one hand you have those who are being cared for by professionals that understand babies, childbirth, and mothers, and who have the utmost respect for the birthing process and a woman's ability to birth her baby. (We need MORE of these people!!)

But there are also a bunch of healthcare professionals who are risk-averse. Perhaps they've only ever seen the worse possible birth outcomes and are keen to avoid them at all costs. Put simply, their goal is to ensure that you birth a baby who is alive. It's less about ensuring that mother and baby have the most positive experience so that mother and baby's well-being is supported for years to come. No - that's YOUR goal. Not theirs. It should be, but sadly it isn't. Their goal is to make sure that you and/or your baby don't die that day. I know this sounds harsh, but there's no point beating around the bush here.

The other consideration that we need to be really clear on is this: money! Depending on where you are in the world, then this will either be:

They want to save themselves unnecessary costs

Typically, this refers to being sued. If anything goes wrong, they run the risk of their department being sued for negligence later. They're less bothered about costs incurred in other departments, though, just ones that show up in THEIR department. So if mum needs mental health support postnatally, well, that's not on their books so it's not a consideration for them. I know this might sound brutal, and of course there are many maternity support professionals who DON'T work like this, but there are also plenty that do. In some countries the system is such that many professionals are forced to work like this, even though they'd rather not. So I simply want you to be aware and take responsibility for your well-being; you can't assume that others are doing this for you. If they are, great! You'll be fine!

They want to make more money

In the US, it makes good business sense to make the birth as medical as possible (drugs, procedures, tests, etc.) because all this can be billed. Watch *The Business of Being Born* if you're keen to understand this a bit better and have your eyes opened. To give you a flavour of the cost differences, in the UK Cesarean sections have been found to cost an average of £2,369 (about US$3,150, while a vaginal delivery costs an average of £1,665 (about US$2,213)[10].

If you want to allow your birth to progress as naturally as possible, then any pressure you experience from your healthcare providers is likely to be tough to deal with. After all, they're the professionals who, you assume, know what they're doing. So it can be quite natural to wonder, "Who the hell am I to go against advice from a medical professional?" but you might have to, for the sake of you and your baby. You are the ONLY one who has both of your long-term interests at heart. I know it sounds crazy, but it's true. I simply want to encourage you to take responsibility for your birth and your baby. Parenting starts now. Take the time well in advance to familiarise yourself with:

- Your rights when it comes to labour and birth
- The risks of various options that might be presented to you
- Any recent research or evidence that may apply to your particular situation

This is so that you can confidently navigate the questions, decisions, and pressures that may come your way, and not feel forced into making a decision from a place of fear, one that you might find hard to live with once the fear has passed and you're able to see the facts in the cold light of day.

What Does Due Date Stress Look Like?

You may have started reading this chapter thinking, "Due date stress? Is this woman crazy? She must be a delicate flower to be stressed out by a due date!" So let me share with you how I came to fully understand and appreciate how stressful the due date can be. But before I do, let me also make it clear that with my first pregnancy, my due date was a non-event. I had a healthy, easy-going pregnancy and my baby was born five days after her due date, so I completely escaped the stress-fest that I'm referring to. I still had a bit of anxiety, because I had started the induction conversations with my midwife, but thankfully my daughter made an appearance before I needed to make any decisions. I wouldn't have said that I experienced stress per se, but if there was any, it was pretty short-lived and easy to deal with. My second pregnancy, however, was a completely different story.

When I had my first meeting with my consultant at twenty weeks, she mentioned that I would be having an induction at thirty-nine weeks due to my advanced maternal age (I would have just passed my fortieth birthday around my due date). My position on inductions was clear; I didn't want one unless there was a medical reason for it, so I knew that I would have to do my homework before my follow-up meeting, which I did. So while I was prepared for my thirty-nine week meeting in terms of the facts, I wasn't prepared for the way I'd be spoken to.

I decided to remain quiet and let the consultant lead the way, out of curiosity. She started with the line " . . . last thing we want is for you to deliver a stillborn" before elaborating by saying that in people like me (old, geriatric types) ". . . the placenta stopped sustaining baby" and that " . . . a stillborn would be traumatic for everyone involved".

Wow! Thankfully I had read every piece of research that I could find on the risks facing women of advanced maternal age, as well as everything I could read on the risks of being induced so I felt confident in asking her to share with me her sources of evidence as this wasn't what I had found. She wasn't able to show me anything, instead she asked to see me again in three weeks (at forty-one weeks) to discuss inductions. Again, wow! Just like that, the induction was off the table and I had an extra three weeks to let my baby cook. This experience demonstrates how far the healthcare professionals would go to coerce me to go down a route of their choosing even if it wasn't the right choice for me and my baby. The importance of me being well informed and educated about the risks was made very clear.

My follow-up meeting was quite unexpected, but not in a good way. My previous meeting was an obvious case of using fear and scaremongering to persuade me to be induced, this time things were conked up a notch. This consultant was much more informed on matters of the latest research; I think she had prepped, knowing I was coming! However, she didn't do this from a place of sharing and caring - instead she demanded that I share my sources of research, right there in the hospital. Thankfully, I had them all on my iPad and was able to show her everything. She then countered by citing some of her own sources of research as to the risks I was facing in what sounded like a game of "my research is better than yours." I asked her if I could read the research she was citing, but she didn't have it at hand. Thankfully, I had an Internet connection and was able to look for the research right there in the meeting. While I was checking, she commented, "I'm not used to dealing with people like you." *What? You mean people who want to be well informed and not be bullied into having a medicalised birth for no justifiable reason?* It was unfortunate for her that her "sources of research" were not coming up on the Royal College of Obstetricians and Gynaecologists (RCOG) website as she had claimed. Thankfully, I had mine in black-and-white in front of both of us.

My stance for resisting an induction was based on what I perceived to be an inaccuracy of my due date. Over the course of my research, I discovered a ton of flaws in the due date calculation system and was able to recalculate my due date based on what I found. I'll be sharing all this with you shortly because, as you'll see from my story, having confidence in your due date is crucial when it comes to being pressured for an induction.

I put forward my case for changing the date on my records by sharing with her the dates I came up with using other calculation methods. She countered by saying that we had a date based on a scan and that those are the most accurate. Well, you'd think so, wouldn't you? But when you find that your due date is revised based on a scan, they often forget to tell you about how it's not actually more accurate.

Ultrasound scan dating

Once you've had your twenty-week scan, you may be given a revised due date based on the scan. In fact, each scan provides your health care providers with an indication as to the developmental stage of your baby. However, it's worth knowing that as your baby grows, the estimates around due dates become more inaccurate. This is for the simple reason that we are all different in size and do not conform to the same growth rates, so as your baby grows, their size is much less accurate for determining foetal age. The inaccuracy of ultrasound scans are estimated[11] to be as follows:

First trimester: +/- 7 days
14 – 20 weeks: +/- 10 days
21 – 30 weeks: +/- 14 days
31 – 42 weeks: +/- 21 days

From this, it's clear to see that those who appear from scans to be "at term" (forty weeks) may in fact be anywhere from thirty-seven to forty-three weeks gestational age.

When we step back and think about this, it makes total sense. As an embryo, there is very little scope for a meaningful difference in size; a cell is a cell is a cell. But as we grow, our genetics start to shape who we are to become. So if our father is super tall, then we might start growing long legs. You get the picture! When we think about it like this, it's obvious to see that not every baby is going to be the same size at forty weeks, and that to base age on size starts to appear like a flakey way to progress. Just look at a classroom of thirteen-year-olds to see how different people can look at the same age.

So when you're being given a "term" date and this is used as the basis for an induction recommendation, you need to find out what scan date they're using so you can come to your own conclusions as to what you feel is a more appropriate due date for you. And don't forget to trust your instincts . . . you know your body and your baby more than anyone.

I'd like to reiterate that it's important to consider your own health and well-being as part of this, as well as that of the baby. What's more important than anything is that you take medical advice and protect your baby from any adverse risks. Everything I've shared with you here is to help you to become better informed so that you can make the choice that feels right for you and your family. But if you experience a pregnancy with complications or if you suffer from medical conditions that require close medical supervision, then you must seek medical advice from the appropriate medical professionals.

The consultant I was battling with was persuading me to have an induction because of my due date, September 20, which had been brought forward based on my twenty-week scan (from September 23). What I found baffling was that she wasn't accepting the revised due date that I had calculated (using other evidence based methods that I'll talk about shortly) taking into account personal factors such as my known conception date and my ovulation cycle. This newer estimated due date was between October 1 and 6. As you can see, that's quite some gap!

When I gently reminded her about the known inaccuracies of ultrasound dates, she acknowledged them but unhelpfully suggested that this could also mean that my real due date could be early September. Well, no, actually! Physically and biologically that wasn't possible; my partner and I were on different continents!

She refused to budge, as did I, so eventually she decided to fetch her boss. When her boss returned with her, it was like chalk and cheese. He was a very gentle, caring soul who reassured me that he only wanted to find a solution that was acceptable to both of us. This was more like it! We then negotiated for a bit before agreeing on a date on which I would accept being induced, October 8. I say *negotiated* because that's what it was. He started by offering a date of October 5, I came back, saying that one of the methods said October 9 as a due date so that was still a bit early for me. This is how we settled on October 8. I accepted this because most of my due dates (using three different evidence based methods) would have passed by this time, but I knew that I could still refuse on that day if I wanted to. However, the caveat was that I would need to be monitored every two days here in the hospital so they could check up on Baby and me to make sure we were doing OK.

I left my appointment happy that I had been able to bat away yet another challenging appointment. I was grateful for my stubbornness, but also grateful for the hours and hours I had spent reading and researching because this gave me confidence in my convictions. I never forgot for one moment that the most important thing was to give birth to a healthy baby, and if Baby was ever under any distress while still inside then I needed to take that seriously. However, if Baby was happy and NOT showing signs of distress, then I was definitely NOT going to put her or him through unnecessary distress by pumping my body full of drugs and tricking my body into starting a natural process. Have you ever tried to start your period early? No! Some things just need to be left alone!

The Importance of Being Informed About Due Dates

Even if you're happy to be induced, it can still be a worrying time. We all have different pregnancy journeys and any delays in Baby's arrival can easily trigger worries or concerns about Baby's well-being as well as your own: *Is everything OK?* It's fair to assume that most women want their baby to arrive when it's ready and not a moment sooner.

Our bodies and our baby will know when this is, so it's important to trust your instincts. But trusting your intuition while simultaneously beating off pressure to be induced is not easy, especially when hormones are messing with your head. What really helps at this point is to be able to *trust* your due date. And I'm sorry to be the one to tell you this, but I'm afraid it's probably the one thing that you CAN'T trust. Why? Because it's probably wrong!

If you remember, earlier I mentioned that as part of my prep research for the meeting with my consultant I'd stumbled across information that I believe every pregnant woman should know to help navigate that last month of pregnancy. I'm going to share it with you, but essentially, the information I discovered had to do with the following:

- The gestational age that healthy babies tend to be born at

when birth is allowed to happen naturally
- The percentage of babies born at thirty-nine weeks, forty weeks, forty-one weeks, forty-two weeks, and forty-three weeks
- The *different* methods we can use to calculate due dates and how the one that is the most widely used is known for being wildly inaccurate
- The risks of induction and how choosing to be induced can kick off a cascade of interventions that are never good for you nor Baby
- The risks of waiting for Baby to come out when he or she is ready, even if that might be at forty-four weeks

Just glancing quickly at this list, it's easy to see why this information would be useful for a pregnant woman to know, especially when most of us will have to deal with the induction question at some point.

Going back to my own pregnancy story, it wasn't going to be long before this new information that I had learned was going to be extremely useful to me. Upon leaving the meeting with the consultant I became quite obsessed with it. But the more I read, the more I realised that something was amiss with my due date. When you're being told that you need to be induced at a certain stage in your pregnancy, it makes sense to know whether you are in fact at the stage in your pregnancy that you're being told you are. Not being one to assume that *everyone else knows what they're talking about*, while also being a graduate of the 'Question Everything' school of thought, I wanted to double-check my actual pregnancy week; I needed to be super sure what week I was in so I could form my own conclusion as to my level of risk. It was while doing this and counting my pregnancy weeks that I realised there was no way I could be at thirty-nine weeks. My partner had been working out of the country, so the conception date was well etched in my head. Once I realised that my due date didn't look right, I decided to dig a bit more into the calculation methods I'd read about, and this was when things started to unravel.

This experience was valuable for me because it helped me realise how much actually rests on the due date. It is used to evaluate so much in a woman's pregnancy and a lot of importance is placed on it, with key decisions being made as a result. And yet the more I read, the less confident I became in my own due date, which was proving to be quite critical for me. I was being pressured to have an induction on my due date, and as far as I was concerned, my due date was in question; I wasn't at the gestational point that they thought I was, so surely I wasn't at the risk they thought I was.

It didn't take me long to figure out that my due date had been calculated using a method that is widely accepted for being inaccurate. Yet frighteningly this is the method that is the most widely used by midwives and doctors. In fact, in using this method, it's possible that my due date could be up to three weeks early. That's a lot! This was pretty major stuff, especially since I was being encouraged to sign up for medical intervention on the basis that we can't risk me being late, when in reality baby might not even be ripe yet, let alone ready to come out.

This situation is not unusual, and women face it all the time. In the two month period around the time I was writing this section of the book, I had three pregnant friends (my only pregnant friends at the time - so 100% of them) who all had questionable due dates. Given how important a due date is in a woman's pregnancy, one would assume that the method used to calculate it would be based on some kind of research or science. You'd think so, right? Hmmm. Well, think again! It's not.

The due date calculation method that's widely used is not based on any evidence, science, or research. Let me say that again, because it's pretty staggering and you'd be forgiven for thinking that I'd made some kind of typo or error. In fact, let me put it in bold too, just to be super sure!

The due date calculation method that's widely used is not based on any evidence, science, or research.

Indeed. So let me tell you more about this.

The Joke That Is Due Dates

The Estimated Due Date (EDD) is one of the biggest lies/disasters/tricks/hoaxes/etc. to affect pregnant women today, and even though people who *should* know better *do* know better, this lie still stands. It's a bit like the whole Santa thing but far more damaging, and because of it you're setting yourself up for a ton of stress in the last month or so of your pregnancy. Stress that for the most part can be avoided.

The most commonly used method to calculate due dates is also the most inaccurate. The due date calculation method widely used by doctors and midwives is based on something called Naegele's rule (named after the obstetrician who devised it, Franz Karl Naegele, 1778–1851), and it goes something like this . . .

Naegele's Rule

According to Naegele's rule, the standard definition for gestational term is 266 days from conception to the date of the baby's birth. This is also defined as 280 days, or forty weeks, from the first day of the mother's last menstrual period (LMP). This definition assumes that the mother ovulates on day fourteen of a twenty-eight-day menstrual cycle. The actual formula used to calculate estimated due date is:

(LMP + 7 days) – 3 months = Estimated Due Date (EDD)

This is the formula that was probably used to give you your due date and is probably the one being used in many online EDD calculators. In fact, Naegele's theory originated from a guy called Hermanni Boerhaave, a botanist, chemist, and physician, who in 1744 came up with a method of calculating the Estimated Due Date (EDD) based upon evidence in the Bible that human gestation lasts approximately ten lunar months.

I don't know about you, but for me, there is so much wrong with that last sentence that when I first read it I choked on my cup of raspberry leaf tea. Considering what's at stake here, this calculation method doesn't inspire confidence in me and here's why:

" . . . based on evidence in the Bible . . . "

1744 is like HOW long ago?! You would think, given how many people have been born since then, that we would have built up a pretty good picture of this whole human gestation thing. You know, maybe even taken the time to take a closer look to see if the assumptions we're using are appropriate. You'd think?!

What makes this unforgivable in my mind is that this rule is not based on scientific or empirical evidence or research. None whatsoever. Not even hundred-year-old scientific research when hospitals were a lot muckier than they are now. No! We're talking about times when women gave birth by candlelight. And even though other evidence based methods existed, they're not being used. Bonkers, I tell you! Can you tell that this makes me mad? But it gets worse . . .

" . . . that human gestation lasts approximately ten lunar months"

Lunar cycles?!! Seriously? OK, let's follow this line of thought and see where it takes us. A quick check online will tell you that there are five different lunar months ranging in length from 27.3 days to 29.5 days, but the one that is widely used is the *synodic* month, which Wikipedia describes as "how long it takes on average to pass through each phase (new, half, full moon) and back again," and which lasts 29.5

days. Having been told that human gestation lasts approximately ten lunar months, then according to my calculations 10 x 29.5 = 295 days. (But it could also be 273 days! But who's counting? Oh yes, your care providers are!)

Now if you recall, Naegele's Rule says that human gestation is 280 days. So, given that ten lunar months gives us 295 days , we're already hitting some problems. Let's look at the math:

295 – 280 = 15 days difference

This is fifteen days LONGER than the 280-day gestation period that is being used and that we've been lead to believe is average. That's more than a two-week difference!

So already, even if you use Naegele's Rule, you've got a two-week slack to add onto your due date. Your due date is not an ESTIMATED DUE DATE but a ESTIMATED BIRTHING MONTH. Those in the know understand this already, but lots of first-time mums don't. The problem we have is that the maternity system we become part of obsesses over the due date, especially those who are pressuring you to have an induction. They regularly forget about the whole birthing month thing and are pretty hung up on due dates. But hang on, I'm not finished:

Twenty-eight-day menstrual cycle

Naegele's rule is based on the idea that our menstrual cycle lasts twenty-eight days. Hands up! Whose cycle DOES NOT last twenty-eight days? Most of you, huh? Thought so. We all know that our menstrual cycles vary in length. I know mine is nearer thirty-four days than twenty-eight days. Do you know what yours is? It's accepted that menstrual cycles can last anywhere from twenty-two to thirty-five days. So if your cycle is NOT twenty-eight days then you need to tweak the formula. For example, if your cycle is thirty-four days, you would need to add six days to your due date (34 – 28 = 6), whereas if your cycle is twenty-six days, you would take two days off (28 – 26 = 2).

Ovulation

Naegele's rule assumes that we ovulate exactly halfway through our twenty-eight-day cycle, fourteen days in. But ovulation is not always halfway through a cycle because it can be affected by things like whether you've recently come off birth control pills, or if you're stressed, ill, or experiencing a disruption in routine. In other words: LIFE! So from this it can be fair to assume that most of us have an ovulation cycle that is probably NOT halfway through the month.

How confident are you in your due date?

Now that we've gone through the teensy-weensy details of Naegele's rule, what is your level of confidence in the date you've been given as your Estimated Due Date? More importantly, has all this been explained to you by your care provider so you can better understand this date they're giving you? When you consider everything I've just shared with you, the due date you've been given has the potential to be up to three weeks off. Mmmm . . . so how do you think this is going to affect your stress levels in that last month? And what about your child-birth outcome?

How to Identify a More Realistic
Due Date

Luckily for us, there are three other methods that exist for calculating due dates. They are based on scientific research and evidence carried out in the last fifty years. Yeehaah for modern science!

I'm sure you're wondering, as I did, why these methods aren't used by prenatal and maternity services everywhere, and I'm afraid I have no answer to that. Research papers, midwifery journals, and various associations all over the world are pretty much in agreement that Naegele's rule is inadequate for calculating due dates, and yet its use continues. Using an alternative method is only available to those who take it upon themselves to educate themselves on these matters.

It's simply not enough to assume that you're being provided with the adequate information from your healthcare provider because you're probably not. It's another one of those instances in which you have to spend your time and effort getting hold of some facts that you trust. This is what I did, and I'm sharing with you what I found. Please feel free to read through the sources of information I've come across (provided in the resource section) so that you too can be confident in what you find out.

My intention here is to highlight areas that you may wish to explore further so that you are completely satisfied with the knowledge you have at your disposal. As I've mentioned quite a bit, I am not medically qualified in matters pertaining to pregnancy and childbirth, but I have an inquiring mind and I'm pretty good at reading. Thankfully, that's all you need to uncover the facts here. Oh, and Internet access helps too!

OK, now back to these other methods for coming up with a more realistic due date. To work out your due date using these methods, you'll need to be armed with certain pieces of information:

1. The start date of your last menstrual period (LMP)
2. Your average cycle length (in days)
3. What number pregnancy you're on (a pregnancy being defined as "a woman who has given birth to an infant, live born or not, weighing 500g or more, or having an estimated length of gestation of at least twenty weeks.")

I've identified three other methods for calculating your due date that are based on research. These methods are shown below:

Nichols, 1985a

First and second pregnancy - Gestation 290 days
LMP + 1 year – 2 months 2 weeks
then +/- as many days as your usual cycle length varies from a
28-day cycle

3rd pregnancy onwards - Gestation 286 days
LMP + 1 year – 2 months 2.5 weeks
then +/- as many days as your usual cycle length varies from a
28-day cycle

Park, 1968

EDD = LMP + 1 year + 14 days – 3 months
Gestation 288 days

Mittendorf, et al., 1990

First and second pregnancy - Gestation 288 days
(LMP – 3 months) + 15 days

3rd pregnancy onwards - Gestation 283 days
(LMP – 3 months) + 10 days

Once you've calculated a due date using the above methods you'll end up with a few dates, thereby giving you a timeframe for when your baby can be expected to arrive. It might well be that your current due date sits quite nicely within this range. Or it might not. To give you an idea as to how these dates might look, I'll share with you my dates.

My due date provided to me by my midwife at the start of my pregnancy was September 23. This was revised to September 20 after my twenty-week ultrasound. When I calculated my dates using the above methods, I came up with September 27, October 3, and October 6. My baby was born on October 5, and according to my midwives, she didn't appear late. Late babies sometimes look pale, wrinkly, or dry, and their skin might be described as leathery. However, my daughter still had lots of vernix covering her and was pinkish in colour. As you can see, in my situation, there was quite a difference between the due dates my healthcare providers were basing their decisions on, and mine. I was grateful for having discovered these additional methods of due date calculation because I was able to feel confident in refusing an induction.

However this pans out for you, it's my intention that with this additional information you feel more confident in navigating the potential demands that might come your way, such as being induced. Remember, though, that these methods are still only guesstimates so you still need to apply common sense to your own situation and stay connected to your baby and his or her movements in those final weeks. If in doubt, then speak to your care provider.

Birth Prep Work

If you're pregnant, then take some time to calculate your revised due dates.

I've put all these methods into a downloadable cheat sheet PDF which you will find in the online resources section that accompanies the book. You can also download a copy by visiting www.fear-freechildbirth.com/blog/due-date-calculation/

What Is LATE Anyway?

One thing that I think is really important to understand is what's meant by "late." It may well be that you are being pressured into induction, when in fact you're not "late," you're simply at the tail end of gestation.

- Term (as in a "normal" and healthy gestation period): from thirty-seven weeks to forty-two weeks
- Post-date: the pregnancy has continued beyond the decided-upon due date (i.e., over forty weeks)
- Post-term: the pregnancy has continued beyond term (i.e., forty-two+ weeks)

The World Health Organization's definition of a 'prolonged pregnancy' is one that has continued beyond forty-two weeks, i.e., one that is post-term. This is all very good, but already assumptions are being made that all babies gestate for the same length of time. From what we know about the human being, one thing we can be sure of is that we don't all adhere to a strict timeline. Just think of the age at which:

- Girls start their periods

- Boys' voices lower
- Women start menopause

None of these arrive according to a fixed timetable, so it seems fair to accept that babies aren't necessarily going to come out according to a fixed timetable. It also seems as though genetic differences can influence the "normal" gestation time. One study[12] found "a familial factor related to recurrence of prolonged pregnancy across generations and both mother and father seem to contribute."

Therefore, if the women in your family tend to give birth at forty-two weeks, so might you. I know that in my mother's line there were a number of forty-three-week gestation pregnancies, and all of them delivered healthy babies. The baby and placenta signal to the mother's body that the baby is mature and ready to be born[13], which in turn starts the intricate and complex process that results in the labour and giving birth. So when I went to see my consultant and she was encouraging me to be induced at thirty-nine weeks, I still had another three weeks of normal, healthy gestation to go. Who was to say that my baby was ready to come out "early," on their schedule?

How to Reduce Due Date Stress

There are two approaches you can take here, but it really depends on where you are in your pregnancy as to which one will work best for you.

If you're in your first or second trimester, then it's easy.

LIE!

Yes - LIE ABOUT YOUR DUE DATE! It might sound a bit harsh, but it's well worth it. Simply add two to three weeks to your due date and relax! At least you can relax knowing that you've successfully pushed aside one of your potential future pregnancy stressors.

If this seems a bit too much for you, then why not be the Queen of Vague: give the month you're due but no specifics. Be careful with this one, though, because some people will push you for an actual date, so you need to have one in mind to get them off your back. If you don't, you'll accidentally give them your real due date and then you'll kick yourself for it as you lie awake one night in your final month as you delete yet another text message from a well-meaning but curious friend.

This is a well-recognised technique to help manage that final month. In fact, the Duchess of Cambridge, Kate Middleton, used it for her pregnancies and was Princess Vague. Despite the pressures of revealing where she was in her pregnancy due to her suffering from morning sickness (and from being a Princess in the public eye) she still managed to keep the due date pretty vague. If she can do it, so can you!

Now, these two approaches might sound a little tongue-in-cheek, but they're definitely worth considering if you want to stay as calm as possible in those final few weeks. I'd like to reiterate that it's important to consider your own health and well-being as part of this, as well as that of the baby. What's most important is that you take medical advice and protect your baby from any adverse risks. What I've shared with you here is to help you to become better informed so that you can make the choice that feels right for you and your family. But if you experience a pregnancy with complications or if you suffer from medical conditions that require close medical supervision, then you must seek medical advice from the appropriate medical professionals.

Chapter Seven

The Childbirth Lies

W here Do We Learn About Childbirth?
Over the course of our lives we absorb a lot of information in such a way that we're not really aware of the things going in. They simply seep into our subconscious through our culture: our friends and family sharing their stories with us, watching films and TV shows, and reading things online or in magazines. The thing is, whatever we "learn" in this way can't really be considered to be reliable in any way. It's a combination of anecdotes, stories made up for effect (film, TV, and fiction books), and dramatic or exaggerated real-life events for headlines. To truly learn about birth, we need to take proactive approach and seek out dedicated books and films that are evidence based and whose intention is to educate, but we're unlikely to stumble across these if we weren't seeking them out.

Some of us are lucky to have had formal education in this area and we hope what we learn in an educational environment would "stand up in court" - well researched and documented, academically accepted ideas, based on science or fact when possible. Yet the educational establishment fails miserably in educating us about birth. When I was in school I was shown a video of woman giving birth on her back and screaming in pain; that is not birth education. That's like helping somebody to understand what driving a car is all about and showing them a car careening out of control, rolling down a bank, and exploding into flames. "Oh yeah! This is driving - isn't it cool? You wanna learn?" *Sure.* This happens to some people. And, yes, driving can be fatal. But for the most part, it's OK, as long as you spend the time learning and preparing before getting behind the wheel of a car. It's like childbirth in that respect.

So where does this leave us? Well, let me ask you this: what do you imagine giving birth to be like?

Exercise

Take a few moments to think about this, and jot down your responses to these questions.

- **Where does it usually happen?**
- **Where else can it happen?**
- **Who's present?** Her partner? Family members? Midwives? Some doctors? Everyone mentioned plus a couple of student doctors? Anyone else?
- **How long does it last?**
- **What position is the woman in?**
- **How does the woman appear?** Relaxed? In pain? Stressed? Anxious? Happy? Laughing? Crying? Screaming? Silent?
- **What's the environment like?** Bright lights? Candles and low lights? Clinical? Busy?

What does that little exercise tell you about your perceptions of birth? Now let me ask you this: where did you get these ideas? What helped you to form your ideas?

- School?
- Movies or TV shows?
- Friends and family sharing their personal experiences?

- Personal experience? Were you present at someone else's childbirth? Your own previous childbirth?
- Books and magazines?
- The Internet?

Let's take a closer look at some of these.

School

When I was around age thirteen, my whole biology class was made to watch a video of a woman giving birth. The birth we were shown was not pretty. In fact, it was pretty horrific; she was on her back screaming, there was blood and bodily fluids everywhere, medical machines all over the place, and it all looked pretty painful and stressful. It was the best contraception they could've hoped for. Come to think of it, there were no teenage pregnancies in my year at school, so maybe that was their plan. That video stayed with me for years; you could say it had a lasting impact, certainly on an emotional level. It instilled in me a real fear of childbirth and labour that only added to the ones that were already buried deep in my subconscious.

Out of all the possible births to show a class of impressionable teenagers, they chose to showcase a particularly negative example. I wonder why that was, since it gave me the impression that this was how childbirth is. Period. There was never any hint that this was just one possible outcome and yet, that is exactly what it was: just one version of the childbirth experience out of a whole spectrum of possibilities. There are also calm, non-scary, peaceful, joyous birthing experiences. While I don't think for one minute that we should only present the positive possibilities, I think it's important to show a balanced view, and that means enabling girls (and boys!) to understand that there are several possibilities when it comes to giving birth, and that choices and variations of normal exist.

Movies & TV shows

If there was ever a possibility that the contraceptive-motivated version of birthing that we were exposed to at school hadn't gotten through, then parents, don't fret! Movies and TV shows are more than happy to pick up where schools leave off and continue propagating the idea that childbirth is a complete and utter nightmare: a hospital room full of unsightly medical outfits and machines, and a heap of screaming women, one of them usually being in obvious pain, while simultaneously being "on display." What's not to like? And don't even get me started on "reality" birthing TV shows!

It's a sad state of affairs that the bulk of birthing education today is through reality birth shows. TV shows that are edited for drama and ratings and whose objective is advertising dollars rather than birthing education. Unfortunately, these shows don't come with a warning; they are presented as reality, which has far-reaching and damaging consequences when it comes to the pregnant women of the future.

Friends & family

Depending on your age, life-stage, and friends, this may or may not be quite a significant source of information for you. If all your friends have had babies and you have lots of female family members then you've probably heard quite a few pregnancy and childbirth stories. Personally, I wasn't in a group of friends that had done or were doing the baby thing when I was pregnant, and there were no women in the family to tell me their own stories. My mother died when I was thirty, an age when having kids was the *last* thing on my mind (probably due to my extreme irrational fear and dread), so we never got the chance to discuss things like kids, pregnancy, and childbirth. But maybe things are very different for you and you've heard quite a few stories. The rest of you are probably somewhere in between.

However, now that I've had children and that I've been among groups of women that have discussed their childbirth experiences, I've noticed this: the negative experiences tend to get a lot more airtime. This probably boils down to our need to get such experiences off our chest and our need for support in recovering from them. Unfortunately, there's also a bit of competitiveness that comes out - my birth was worse than yours, etc. - as women vie for the bravery award in their social group.

The unfortunate side effect of this is that the positive birth stories often get brushed aside. Just as our newspapers are mostly filled with bad news - the more terrifying and scaremongering the better - positive, happy stories just don't sell papers in the same way! For my podcast, I've interviewed many women about their positive birth experiences and a lot of them tell me that this is the first time that they've shared their birth experience. I've even observed and been told about countless situations wherein some positive birth stories have been interrupted with comments such as, "Yeah, that's great. Anyway . . . how IS the little one?" Perhaps this happens because the negative birthing experiences that may have occurred for those listening are simply too painful and they'd rather not hear a positive version. This too is a sad sign that women aren't able to get the support they need to get over the negative birthing experiences.

Personal experience

If you've ever attended someone else's birth, this is likely to be very clear in your mind due to the inevitable emotional intensity of the experience. When we experience strong emotions during an incident, it is more likely to stay with us, if not in our conscious mind, then certainly in our subconscious. This means that it also has the ability to influence how we feel about the future occurrence of such incidents. It therefore follows that if you've been present at a positive birthing experience, it's from this perspective that you will perceive future birthing experiences.

If your personal experience is a previous time that you have given birth then you know first-hand what childbirth is like and it will influence how you think about childbirth, depending on how that went for you. However, even though you may have given birth previously, it's important to maintain an open mind. Childbirth experiences vary wildly, and a past experience is no indication of a future one. So if you've had a difficult previous birth, there is no reason to assume that it will be repeated. Just as if you had a wonderfully positive one, there's no reason to expect this to be repeated.

Books, blogs, magazines

There are plenty of great resources available to us if we want to learn more about childbirth. However, generally speaking, these require us to seek out positive information. It's unlikely that that you will simply stumble across a balanced, in-depth resource on childbirth unless you seek it out, and you're unlikely to seek it out unless you're pregnant and it suddenly becomes relevant for you. So while this information is readily available, it doesn't readily find its way into our hands. The stuff that you're more likely to stumble across are the headline-grabbing stories that get picked up by the mass press, and headline-grabbing stories don't usually include things along the lines of "Mother has peaceful, joyous birth at home with no fuss."

Social media

If you're active on social media then this will also be a source of information for you. Your Facebook feed will be based on the pages you like, the friends you're connected to and the things you tend to click on. If you're seeing birth negativity in your feed there are some simple steps you can take to change the information you're exposed to. Start liking pages that educate, inform and inspire when it comes to birth. You can choose to unfollow certain friends who constantly share information that doesn't support you. Once you do this, it won't take long for you to start being exposed to sources of information that will support you during your pregnancy.

What Are We Being Told About Childbirth?

It's possible that your impression of childbirth is that it happens in a hospital, with a woman on her back surrounded by lots of medical staff, and that it looks like she's having tough time. It's a sad fact of our times that many women think this. If you didn't, then hip-hip-hoorah!! You probably know that birth can happen just as safely at home or in a birthing centre, and that the woman can be walking about, crouching, or in water during her birth. She might even be at home with candles and soft music playing. And *NEWSFLASH* she might even be happy, relaxed, and enjoying herself! Crazy, right? That a woman giving birth could actually be having one of the most powerfully positive and spiritual moments of her life and be LOVING IT!

Where are these versions of birth? How come we don't see birthing moments like these reveal themselves through the media and with conversations with friends and family? Good question! Instead, we are fed a cocktail of negativity and drama around birth that only represents a tiny proportion of how birth can be. The problem with this is that it acts as a self-fulfilling prophecy. There are some consistent themes that we're being fed, themes that aren't exactly accurate. But worse than that, these are communicated as *truths*. So what are they?

- Labour and childbirth WILL be painful. Excruciatingly painful. This seems to be a given, and non-negotiable.
- Childbirth is a medical situation. This is why most babies are born in hospitals, right?
- Childbirth requires medical assistance. Childbirth needs an army of nurses and doctors to be present, as well as some scary-looking medical machines and instruments. And the woman giving birth is going to need a whole host of medical aids - epidural injections, forceps, etc.
- Women give birth on their backs. It's just the way it is, right?

When you look at these in the cold light of day, it's all too easy to understand why so many women are fearful of birth. If women grow up to believe that birth is going to be this highly painful experience in which she's in a vulnerable position on her back with strangers looking at her wotsit, is it any surprise that so many women fear it?

Many women (and men) want children, and yet the main thing that stands between them and being parents is the birth. So while sex is something we can all get excited about, childbirth isn't. Sadly, as I shared in my chapter on tokophobia, many women choose not to have children because of their fear of childbirth. So should we be actively feeding this fear? Should we be ALLOWING the flames of this fear to be fanned? Given how fear can impact birth outcomes, I'd say NO!

Childbirth experiences are sacred

What I'd like us to realise is that by perpetuating these lies about birth, we're feeding into a powerful psychological loop that impacts women's birthing experiences. Childbirth experiences are sacred and we need to do everything we can to protect them as much as possible. The birthing experience doesn't only affect the mother; it affects the whole family for years to come. A traumatic birth affects everyone in the family, even the dads! Many fathers report experiencing PTSD as a result of seeing their children born. Here are just some of the ways that a family can be affected by the birthing experience:

- Mother-baby bonding
- Breastfeeding success
- How the mum feels about the birth and how that affects her forever
- How the baby experienced it and how that will impact their future physical, emotional, and mental well-being
- How dads feel about the birth

What's so sad about all of this is that as women we have been conditioned since our school days to think that childbirth is not something we can do on our own, but something we *need help with*. Medical help. On the one hand, our biology lessons taught us that women (not men) are built to conceive and give birth to ensure the survival of our race, and yet popular culture bombards us with messages that lead us to believe that actually, we're not really capable of doing what our bodies were built to do. In fact, we're just not good enough - we're failures!

But there's a double-whammy here. The more we are fed the myth that childbirth requires medical assistance, the less likely we are to *believe* that it's a natural process that can happen perfectly adequately on its own. Of course, there are still risks, as with most things in life - risks that are increased if the health of the mother is compromised, or if she doesn't have access to adequate healthcare. So in developing countries, childbirth brings with it a more increased risk than it does for those of us in developed countries. But that is not what I'm talking about here. I'm talking about helping women to believe that they can do this on their own. That they are enough. That they have everything they need within them, and for this to be the starting point.

We need to stop perpetuating these lies about birth so women can have a chance at having a positive birthing experience that empowers them and brings joy to their families for years to come. In helping women to have a positive birthing experience, we're helping families to experience better bonding and we're contributing to positive well-being. Who knows how this could impact society as a whole? The childbirth experience is a pivotal moment in everyone's lives. No one escapes it. We need to protect it fiercely. So how do we do that?

Given the media's influential role in shaping women's views on birth, we need to start there. This is one reason why I started my *Fear Free Childbirth* podcast. It was my hope that I could at least start to tip the balance the other way, one listener at a time. At the time of this writing, I have over 300,000 downloads under my belt, so I have a sense that I'm making a difference. But it's only a ripple compared to the daily tsunami of myth-perpetuating media messages.

It's certainly worthwhile to contribute to the grassroots movement that exists around positive childbirth, but why not take a double-pronged approach? I figured, let's go to the source. We need to effect change among the mass media publishers. So I thought I'd target those who televise the *enfant terrible* of bad-birth PR in the UK. I decided to start a petition against the TV network who broadcasts *One Born Every Minute*, Channel 4.

My petition on Change.org was this: *Ask Channel 4 to portray childbirth in a more balanced way as part of their programming.*

Why I started the petition

It all started after I spoke to a TV producer who was developing a TV series that aimed to show the "other" side of birth and she was looking for positive birth stories to share. During the course of our conversation it transpired that Channel 4 had said that they wouldn't be interested in taking a whole series from her, just one episode. "Just the one?" I asked. Yes. So they're happy to relentlessly promote a narrow medical view of birth that instills fear in women, but they're not interested in also showing women the alternatives when it comes to birth? Mmm. This annoyed me.

I get it. They're in the business of entertainment, not education. Unfortunately, as we've just learned, due to the lack of effective education for young women (and dads-to-be) when it comes to childbirth, TV is filling the void. So we find ourselves in a situation in which most people are looking to a reality TV show that represents a narrow medical view of birth, which is edited for drama and effect, to better understand what birth is all about. And it's this that is forming the mainstay of childbirth education across the Western world. How tragic, sad, and pitiful.

When my petition hit the press, I got a lot of crap on social media. After all, it appeared on the surface that I was taking aim at everybody's favourite TV show. Headlines such as "Mum wants to ban *One Born Every Minute*" didn't help. Anyone who took to time the read the actual petition could see that I was not actually calling for a ban. But newspapers rarely report the facts; they seek out the drama to sell clicks and copies. Let me repeat, I am not looking to ban the show. What I'm seeking is for media owners to portray birth in a more balanced way and to accept the responsibility that comes with their programming forming an integral part of childbirth education. They might not like where they've found themselves, but now that they're there, they need to put on some big-girl pants and act responsibly. So if a TV producer approaches them to offer a series exploring the positive side of birth, then they should show it or something similar.

A lot of my social media trolls were keen to point out how much *One Born Every Minute* helped them to prepare for their birth. Interestingly, it also transpired that for many of them, this was a good thing because their birth didn't go that well. But at least they were prepared! Is it just me, or is there an obvious pattern here?

On the other hand, if you spend time with mums that have had beautiful, calm, and joyous births, one thing stands out as being consistent: NONE of them watch shows like *One Born Every Minute*. Instead, they proactively seek out positive birth stories and videos or films online showing calm, peaceful births. Many midwives, doulas and hypnobirthing teachers tell their pregnant mamas to AVOID watching the show while pregnant.

I believe we should be spreading the following truths instead:

Childbirth doesn't have to hurt

If you surrender to the process and let nature do her thing, it doesn't have to. The whole thing about pain in childbirth is quite interesting. It's so interesting and worth understanding that I dedicate a whole chapter to it (the next one!). So if you're about to throw this book at the wall in disbelief, hold your horses. I'm not kidding: childbirth doesn't have to hurt. Not only will I explain why, but I'll help you to get closer to it being possible for you.

Childbirth is not an illness or a medical condition

This means that it does not require doctors or a hospital by default. It only becomes a medical condition if Mum's health is compromised or the baby is in distress. But for the most part, it's a natural process that happens much more safely and with better outcomes at home. If your dog or cat was pregnant, would you take them to the vet to birth their little ones? Probably not, because that would be weird. You'd just let them find their quiet spot behind the sofa or wherever they're most comfortable.

Childbirth does not require medical assistance

Childbirth is a natural process that can happen quite happily on its own. It does not require drugs, injections, or medical equipment to have a positive outcome. It only needs those things if complications arise, and they are more likely to arise if the natural birthing process has been interrupted in some way, say because you've been induced. An induction often leads to what is known as the cascade of interventions, which ultimately might lead to an emergency C-section. If you create the space to allow nature to be in control and to set the pace, then no medical interventions should be required. Unless, of course, complications arise - so then, yes, it's hands-off: let the medical teams do their thing!

You can birth how the hell you want!

In fact standing up and moving around will help to make the whole thing easier. But if you fancy lying down, then do that. Many women hear about the things they're "allowed" to do during labour. Well, know this; being "allowed" doesn't even come into it. You have the right to do what you want. If you are being told that you're now allowed to do something, then challenge it.

**It's your body, your baby, your birth.
YOU decide!**

Sure, suggestions can be made. And they might be very good suggestions, but you have the final say. Getting savvy about birth and your rights will help you to navigate this treacherous terrain and feel confident in standing up for what you want.

Chapter Eight

Childbirth and Pain

Unfortunately, *childbirth* and *pain* are two words that are often used hand-in-hand. This is a real shame because this alone adds to a lot of the fear that women have about birth. Sure, some people experience pain in childbirth, but some don't. It's not a given that childbirth *will* be painful, more that it *might* be.

Having a fear of pain is something I am completely familiar with because it was one of my biggest fears during my first pregnancy. During my first trimester I was of the opinion that *childbirth is the most painful thing ever* and that I was going to demand all the drugs I could get my hands on to get me through my labour and childbirth. I didn't know otherwise at that point and I just couldn't see how I was going to get through this. *What if I can't cope? What if I have a total meltdown?*

For me, this all changed the day that Julie, an acquaintance, told me that birth could be natural while being painless and enjoyable. She went on to say that the secret was hypnobirthing. Hypnobirthing is the use of hypnosis to make childbirth easier. Or at least it was when it started; it's broadened its scope and is now considered to be a holistic approach to birthing preparation that includes self-hypnosis, but also things like childbirth education, visualisation, positive affirmations, breathing techniques, and involving your birth partner.

Once I discovered hypnobirthing, I devoured everything I could about it. If a natural, pain-free birth was possible, then I wanted it. But more than that, I was curious:

How on earth is it possible NOT to experience pain during childbirth?

What was that all about? Given that fear of pain was one of my biggies, I really needed to get my head around this, so that's what I did.

I spent more time than I'd care to admit reading about pain. The thing is, once I started, I kept having to go back for more because pain is actually quite an interesting subject and not as clear-cut as you might think. I've also got this nerdy thing going on where I like to simplify stuff and distill it down to its essentials. I'm not one for wasting headspace with useless fluff. So naturally I did this with what I learned about pain. For me, it all came down to this: there are three things that pregnant mamas need to understand about pain in order for them to overcome their fear of it.

Let me share with you what those three things are.

Pain is All in The Mind

PAIN CONCEPT #1

Pain is subjective; not everyone experiences it in the same way or to the same degree. We know this from how people around us respond to painful experiences. Pain clearly involves a physical sensation, but what we probably don't acknowledge enough is that the experience of pain also inherently involves unpleasant and distressing thoughts, feelings, and behaviours that just *add* to the pain; emotional pain, if you will. So from that perspective, pain is essentially a construct of the mind.

Over the last few years scientists have begun to realise that pain, which is processed in many of the same areas of the brain as stress, fear, and anxiety, is as much an emotional as a sensory experience. This means that it's often held up as being symbolic of what can be achieved (or not!) once you master the mind-body connection. I love this because it means that the whole pain thing is up for grabs!

Pain researchers from Stanford[14] are now saying that our experience of pain is spread across two parts of the brain; the first that handles the sensory input (whether you're experiencing a cut, heat or stabbing, for example) and the second is handling the emotional aspect of the pain (how you feel about it).

What's interesting about pain is that it's often made worse by two things:

1. Anticipation of it
2. Fear and avoidance of it

Anticipating pain increases its likelihood and intensity

If we imagine we are going to experience pain, we will. It's a self-fulfilling prophecy. To better understand the dread of pain, an interesting study[15] was carried out by Giles Story and his colleagues at University College London. They hooked up thirty-three volunteers to a device that gave them mild electric shocks. The researchers also presented the participants with a series of choices between more or less painful shocks, and whether they wanted them sooner or later. The research team was able to figure out that the dread of pain increased exponentially as pain approached in time. They achieved similar results in a test using hypothetical dental appointments. This demonstrates that the fear that arises from the anticipation is something in its own right. From this it would be fair to say that much of our pain in life come from the anticipation of a future event or from the memory of a past event, rather from the actual experience we're facing. This is pretty much what George Loewenstein, a professor of economics and psychology at Carnegie-Mellon University in Pittsburgh, Pennsylvania, says[16] on the matter anyway.

Fear and avoidance of pain increases its likelihood

Fear and anxiety in regards to pain increases the likelihood of it being experienced, and when it IS experienced, it's worse than it would have been had we not been fearful or anxious. But it doesn't stop there. There's another aspect to pain that's particularly relevant for those of us about to give birth: a direct physiological relationship between fear and pain. Yes, fear creates pain. So the more fearful you are, the more pain you will experience. This all boils down to what is widely known as the Fear-Tension-Pain Cycle, which is particularly relevant when the area that may be affected by pain is a muscle (e.g., affected by tension). As labour and childbirth requires your uterus - your largest muscle by mass - to dilate the cervix to help Baby down the birth canal, then this is definitely something we should be looking at more closely.

The Fear - Tension - Pain Cycle

The Fear-Tension-Pain (FTP) Cycle was discovered in the 1930s and goes like this: when there is fear, the body tenses, and when there is fear and tension, pain is amplified. So when there is fear and tension in childbirth, the pain of the contractions seems more intense than it truly is.

When a person is in fear, their state of mind triggers the body into the fight-or-flight stress response. When the body is in this state, it's flooded with adrenaline to help the person either to escape (run away) or fight. As such, the body tenses up and blood is sent to the extremities (legs and arms) to help with the fight-or-flight response. This state is meant to be used sparingly by the body, as the body suffers when it's subject to this level of stress for prolonged periods.

Let's imagine for a minute you live in rural Australia and you're coming up to your due date. You and your partner decide to head out for a walk into the bush for a big dose of nature. Suddenly, labour kicks in much earlier than you had anticipated! So you find a nice spot under a tree. Things start happening quite quickly, but your man spots a croc and says you've got to run. In a flash, your body shifts from *squeezing-out-baby* mode to *run-like-the-wind* mode. That humungous uterine muscle of yours that's been squeezing the little bean out decides that now is not a good time and tightens up pronto. All your blood diverts from your uterus to your legs so that you can scoot off at high speed to ensure you and your baby's survival. You just about make it back to the ute in one piece. Phew! That was close! You're panting like crazy, your adrenaline is pumping through your body, and you're feeling mighty stressed. At this point your lady wotsit is now well and truly shut tight.

So, how do you think it would feel to go against nature at this point and force your body to push the little bean out? It would hurt, that's what! Our body's stress response hasn't changed from the times when sabre tooth tigers roamed the earth, and it doesn't distinguish between real life-threatening danger and imagined danger in the form of fear. Even if your life isn't being threatened, but you experience fear, the stress response is the same: the body tenses and blood gets diverted from major organs to the extremities. While you're in a state of fear and stress, your body doesn't feel safe enough to allow labour to unroll at full pelt, so it slows it down, if not stops it altogether. Two to three days of labour anyone? Guess what's happened there: fear and stress has slowed labour right down, perhaps to a halt.

So why does stress stop labour? Ah, my lovelies. That is the final thing you need to understand about pain and childbirth: the delicate dance of your hormones!

The Delicate Dance of Your Hormones

If you're a woman reading this, I imagine you have a pretty good idea of how powerful your hormones are. But if you're in any doubt, then their ability to completely transform your personality and state of mind every month should be enough to sway you. So it should come as no surprise that these highly strung disrupters of our life take centre stage when it comes to childbirth, in a magical dance that relies on them achieving a very precise yet delicate balance. Each one has a clear role to play and knows exactly when they need to show up to weave their magic. The problem with this tightly knit performance is that the performers are easily knocked off balance, and when that happens, the whole show comes crashing down. Let me introduce to you the hormonal cast of the childbirth show:

Oxytocin

Oxytocin is sometimes referred to as the pleasure or the love hormone. It's present during lovemaking. Ha! I used that word over sex, because it's the great kind of sex that involves love as opposed to the other types of sex. (In case you're wondering, the lust hormone that's present when passions run high is neutrophin). Oxytocin is the hormone that triggers labour and keeps it progressing, ultimately resulting in the birth of Baby. Unfortunately, oxytocin is a bit shy and delicate. So it only feels like coming out to play when you're in an environment that makes you feel safe, secure, and private. (Unless you're an attention-seeking extrovert who would feel totally OK with having sex in the middle of the football field at half time, say.) For oxytocin to flow, you need to feel safe, secure, and loved. If you feel vulnerable or exposed, then it'll stay away. Think about that when it comes to planning the environment for your birth.

Endorphins

Endorphins are the body's natural pain killers and are more effective that anything man-made. What makes them so damn amazing is that not only do they alleviate pain (brilliantly), but they also promote feelings of love and happiness. They're pretty miraculous, actually, because they create the physical sensations of pleasure (sex again!) and are responsible for the feelings of euphoria that come from exercising. So whether it's the post-sex rush or the post-run buzz, endorphins are the little fellas that you can thank for that amazing feeling.

Adrenaline

Adrenaline can be thought of as the stress hormone, and it's the one responsible for triggering the fight-or-flight response in your body. When you're stressed, your adrenal glands release a load of adrenaline into your body. The adrenaline diverts blood away from your main organs to your extremities so that you can defend yourself or run away. Adrenaline is quite a powerful hormone, and a bit of a bully, to be honest. When adrenaline shows up, oxytocin and endorphins usually scamper. Think about that for a minute.

When labour is progressing nicely, your body is flooded with oxytocin and endorphins, each working together as nature intended to help your body give birth to a new life. Oxytocin keeps the show on the road while endorphins work hard to make the journey pleasurable and pain-free. But if something happens to rock your boat and you lose that safe, private feeling, the stress you feel in that moment, no matter how minimal, will send adrenaline flooding in like an Indian monsoon. As soon as that happens, the oxytocin and endorphins get washed away. No oxytocin means that labour slows down (if not stops altogether), and the best pain relief known to humankind vanishes. What do you think that's going to do to your childbirth experience?

Well, it's going to drag on and on and on, and it's going to hurt like crazy. In fact, if you put those two things together, it doesn't take Sherlock to figure out why women turn to epidurals and C-sections. No wonder so many women have horrific births. Once I understood this, it was pretty clear to me what I needed to do. I had to minimise the stress, if not banish it entirely, so that oxytocin and endorphins could do their thing. I wanted nature on my side to enable me to bring my baby into the world in the most magically wonderful way I could, for both Baby's benefit and my own.

Understanding the interplay of these hormones was incredibly liberating and motivating. I realised in that moment how it could be done; I just had to do it. I'm not saying that the journey to a stress-free pregnancy and a fear-free birth is an easy one. But if you're up for it, then it is possible.

The Secret to Minimising Pain in Childbirth

OK, so we've had a whirlwind tour of pain, but what does it all mean when it comes to labour and childbirth? And more importantly, how is all this going to help you experience less of it on the Big Day?

First of all, we learned from some pain experts over at Stanford that pain is all in the mind. The important things they highlighted were:

1. Anticipation of it *increases* the likelihood of us experiencing it, or makes our experience of it *worse*.
2. Fear of pain also has the same effect: it increases the likelihood of us experiencing it, or makes whatever experience we're having even worse.

These two snippets are terribly interesting to me, especially when we cast our minds back to how society and popular culture condition us when it comes to childbirth.

"Childbirth is PAINFUL!"

The idea that childbirth will be painful is regularly reinforced throughout our lives and there's not much escape from it. Births in TV and in the movies always look like complete and utter nightmares:

Midwives are screaming "PUSH! PUSH! PUSH!" Mothers are on their backs screaming in pain. As if that wasn't enough, we have all those birthing horror stories that other women are more than happy to share with us the minute we're pregnant. No wonder we think that the whole giving birth thing is going to be excruciating.

The thing is, as we know from what we've already covered in this book, the very idea that we think it will hurt means it will hurt more than if we didn't think that. So it follows that if we stop imagining and fearing that it will hurt and be painful, it won't be. Now, I know what you're thinking: "Hang on a minute, Lex! Are you crazy?! You can't just make that level of pain go away with positive thinking!"

Well, let me invite you to consider the possibility that yes, we can. Let me show you how.

How to Reduce Your Experience of Pain

What I'm going to share with you here is exactly the approach I took and that I teach to my fearless mamas. Now, the great thing about this approach is that it's not reserved for childbirth. You can apply it to anything, but for now I'll stay focussed on the whole childbirth thing.

Step 1: Don't anticipate the pain

Imagining that you will experience pain makes it more likely to happen. You're basically conditioning your body into a response. If you want to reduce pain, simply don't anticipate that you will experience pain.

If you've already given birth and experienced it as extreme pain, then I imagine you might find this hard. But I'm not asking you to go back and remember a past experience - I'm asking you to wipe your slate clean and consider a whole new childbirth experience that does not involve experiencing pain. Pain isn't an automatic experience for everyone when it comes to birth, so remain open to the possibility that this could include you. This won't guarantee that you won't experience pain, but it will help to reduce your experience of it and how you feel about it.

Remember what the Stanford scientists said: our anticipation or memory of something is often more painful that the actual experience. And they're from Stanford! They know their shizzle!

Step 2: Visualise a pain-free experience

As you spend time visualising your labour and birth, be sure to let your body know that this will be a pain-free experience so your body will be more likely to cooperate and reduce the pain you do experience. So as you think about your upcoming birth, focus your attention on how easy you'll find it, how powerful it will feel, and how smoothly it will go for you. Remember, this is your imagination and you are in total control as to what you decide to come up with in your head. Deciding to imagine your future experience as painful is just silly; why would you do that? Don't fool yourself into thinking that imagining the pain in advance is all part of your necessary preparation because it's not. This kind of thinking is more likely make it happen.

Remember, if you've already given birth and experienced extreme pain, I'm asking you to imagine a future experience instead of focussing on your past experience. These are very different mental exercises. When you spend time visualising, keep your mind focussed on imagining a future experience and not clouding your thoughts with traces of your past. When you think about a holiday you're about to go on, I'm guessing that you get really excited imagining how great your holiday is going to be, not remembering a past holiday that was a disaster and imagining that your future holiday is going to go the same way. So why would you do this when it comes to your birth?

Step 3: Clear your fear of pain

If you are fearful of pain, then this needs to be cleared. I will show you how to clear your fears later on, so if this is on your list of fears, make sure you add it to your list. If the thought of pain scares you, I urge you to work on two aspects of pain: first, make friends with it, and then work on clearing your fear of pain. Once we can make friends with pain - accept it, love it, be OK with it - then we are less likely to fear it. So in the interests of being super thorough, this is what I recommend.

** SHORTCUT **

I've created a *Fearless Birthing Fear Clearance Meditation* to address this fear, so if you'd prefer to just sit back and let me do the clearance work, then visit: www.fearfreechildbirth.com/product/fear-of-pain/

Step 4: Seek out evidence of positive, pain-free experiences

This is quite an important step. By finding evidence that a pain-free experience is possible, you can support your belief that it's possible to reduce pain if not eliminate it completely, as well as super-charge your visualisation work. Many of the positive birthing experiences that I share on my podcast have women saying they didn't experience pain, so be sure to check them out. These stories aren't rare; you'll find plenty of them in the positive birth Facebook groups as well as on blogs.

I interviewed the author of *Painless Childbirth*, Giuditta Tornetta, on my podcast and you might find what she has to say quite useful as you imagine your upcoming birth. To listen to it, just visit www.fear-freechildbirth.com/blog/giuditta-tornetta-painless-childbirth/

Now, I'd just like to say this again because it is important: doing all of these things will not guarantee a pain-free experience, but they will definitely help you get much closer to one. Many women who have done this have told me that they didn't consider their birth painful. Intense? Yes! But the sensations they experienced weren't considered painful. Right at the beginning of the book, when I was talking about hypnobirthing and how they don't like the word pain. Well this is because pain is an emotionally loaded word that carries baggage. If you let go of the emotion around a word, then its use no longer bothers you. This is what's going on here.

If and when it comes time for your childbirth and you do experience pain, don't be hard on yourself. It is a hugely demanding experience both physically and emotionally, so if pain ends up being part of your experience just accept it and don't blame yourself or, heaven forbid, think you failed at birth. That is not what this is about. There is no right way to birth.

Feeling intense physical sensations during birth is completely normal. I experienced completely overwhelming and intense physical sensations during birth, but I didn't consider them to be painful. My baby was coming out; of course it was going to be intense. Childbirth is intense on every level: it's powerful, overwhelming, magical, spiritual, joyous, exciting. All of those things are experienced at top whack. That's what makes it so incredible.

Embrace it! Don't fear it.

Chapter Nine

Making Your Birth Choices

M aking choices about your birth is an important milestone that warrants time and effort. There is no right way to birth: there is only what is right for you and your baby at that moment in time. Just because you spend time and effort during your pregnancy in planning your birth doesn't mean that you will be blessed with the outcome you desire, but it will certainly help you to get closer to it. I'm all for winging it in day-to-day life, but birth is one area in life where this is definitely the worst strategy. You are going to be faced with a multitude of decisions that will involve a lot of weighing things up, and some of them won't be easy decisions because of their importance and potential impact. Things like:

- Should I accept the offer of a sweep on my due date?
- What if I want a home birth? What if I want pain medication; then what?
- Do I have to accept the routine IV and foetal monitoring that I see on labour wards?
- Can I just ask for an epidural from the outset?
- Is there a birth pool at the hospital if I want one?

Many decisions about birth choices will involve weighing the risks, so you need to be comfortable with the decisions you're making, because these are things that you will need to live with. If you don't spend the time thinking these things through while you have the time and space, you may end up feeling pressured to make decisions during labour that you just don't feel well-enough informed about. It can be easy to trust the doctors, consultants, and midwives and just go with what they recommend, but they don't always have your and Baby's long-term interests in mind, despite us assuming they do. Of course, many do and are fabulous sources of support, but you will feel much more confident going into your birth if you are well informed. Being forced to making choices without being fully informed can lead women to feel out of control about their birth. Feeling out of control is a key factor in many women's negative birth experiences so taking steps to avoid this is crucial.

Your birth preferences (birth plan)

I prefer to call it a *birth preferences* or *choices* document rather than a *birth plan*, because "plan" feels like a solid thing that's quite precise and can't be changed. Birth is a highly complex event and there is so much potential for things to happen that might take us off plan. So if something does happen that means that we can't have the birth in our plan, we shouldn't feel that we have failed. Citing *preferences* or *choices* is simply another way of thinking about it that doesn't set you up for feeling like you've failed your plan, because this is needless guilt that no one needs in their lives.

At the end of the day, it's all about language and what you feel works best for you, so be mindful as to what you want to call it. If you feel strong and are clear that you will stand your ground no matter what, then *birth plan* may work well for you. But, if *birth plan* feels too strong, then go with *birth choices* or *birth preferences*. Remember that there will be certain aspects to your birth you might feel are non-negotiable - skin-to-skin contact, delayed cord clamping, etc. - whereas other elements might have more flexibility. For example, you might prefer to decline pain relief in thinking about your birth in advance, but on the Big Day, you can reserve your right to change your mind. The important thing here is that you're not setting yourself up to fail. With the things that you can control, do what you can to help you to feel as positive as possible, before, during, and after birth.

Even though I've clearly stated that there is no right way to birth, when I was considering my birth choices, I was very clear in my own criteria in terms of what was important to me:

A positive experience for me

I wanted a positive birthing experience that would fill me with joy every time I thought of it. I would be reminded of it every year, so I wanted it to be a positive memory. I was also aware of the probable link between the childbirth experience and the likelihood of me experiencing postnatal depression, so it was important for me to do everything I could to minimise that possibility by seeking and working towards a positive birthing experience.

To improve my chances of a positive birthing experience, these are some of the things I knew that I wanted to be able to do:

- To have the freedom to move during birth so that I could birth in the way my body wanted to and would feel most comfortable.
- To have access to pain management methods that weren't medical, namely water. So baths, showers, and a birthing pool.
- To be able to eat and drink as I fancied.
- To feel safe, secure, and relaxed.
- To have continuity of care throughout my labour and childbirth (the same midwives throughout, not different people coming in and out).

I also knew that I wanted access to medical services if I needed them. But I wanted to go into my birthing experience not assuming that: you get what you focus on!

A positive experience for my baby

One aspect that I don't feel is considered enough is how the birth will impact the baby, both physically and emotionally. For a long time, hospital staff seem to have forgotten that babies are mini-humans who feel pain and experience emotions, and this has been reflected in how babies are treated on arrival: like they won't remember what happened, or that they won't understand what was said. We now know these assumptions to be wrong, and the way we treat babies on their arrival needs to take the baby's thoughts and feelings into consideration. The environment in which the baby arrives can have a huge impact on how the baby will feel once they're born; things like lighting, noise levels, and human interactions need to be considered from the point of view of the baby. The baby has also just been through an incredibly demanding physical and emotional experience, so we need to consider what's best for them during this momentous event too.

When we look at birth through the eyes of the baby, these are the kind of things that your baby is likely to want:

- Mother feeling confident in her ability to birth her baby and trusting her body to do so safely
- Mother feeling like her baby knows what they're doing and will help her
- No drugs or pain medication that can enter baby's bloodstream or the placenta
- Low lighting and noise levels in the arrival room
- Skin-to-skin contact with Mother straightaway
- No disruption to the umbilical cord while Baby is still drawing blood and oxygen from the placenta
- Reassuring sounds and language from Mother and Father, as well as other people present; no flippant comments about their body or their mode of arrival

- No rough handling of the baby: to wipe them down or weigh them, for example; and certainly no horrible, cold, metal weighing scales or hard surfaces

Safe

It feels silly writing this down, because #DOH of course I want it to be safe for me and my baby, but incredibly there are some people who think that mothers are these selfish beings who choose a certain type of birth for selfish reasons. So that last sentence is for them. Hello! *waves*

Everything I've written above assumes that the birth is going normally, and there's no reason to assume otherwise, unless you've had a problematic pregnancy or have a condition that is known to affect birth outcomes.

If I had to summarise, I'd say this: I wanted an experience that would be as positive as possible for both me and my baby, not just on the Big Day, but over the long-term in terms of both of our well-being. When I say "well-being," I'm referring to both mental and emotional well-being. What I wanted to avoid more than anything was a traumatic experience that would scar me or my baby, mentally or emotionally, for years to come. Once I'd considered the things that were important for me, and weighed that against how my pregnancy had been going, it was clear what kind of birth I wanted: a natural home birth.

Quick reality check here! There's no way I would have been able to even contemplate this as an option when I was still fearful. I was only able to do once I had cleared my fears.

Natural Birth

Before I go any further, I would like to clarify what I mean by a "natural birth" as it is a term that is not the same for everyone. For me, a natural birth is a birth that happens *as nature intended* and *at nature's pace*. This means allowing the body to go into spontaneous labour and then allowing the body to birth without any medical intervention.

Based on everything I had read, I felt that a natural birth was one of the things I could do to offer my unborn child the best start in life: good health and emotional resilience. These things were important to me. They won't be important to everyone, or perhaps they are, but not everyone is willing to do what it takes to maximise their chances of being healthy and enjoying high levels of well-being. We know this from seeing all those people who eat badly, smoke and drink excessively, and don't exercise. What we want and what we do to help us get the thing we want don't always add up.

I realise that by choosing to aim for a natural home birth, it doesn't mean that 1) I will get it, and 2) it will turn out that way. Just as we cannot guarantee that offering our children a good education will mean that they will 1) pass their exams, and 2) go on to lead a happy, successful, and meaningful life. But that doesn't mean we shouldn't try do everything we can to maximise the likelihood of the outcome we have in mind.

Of course, there are other things that we can do as expectant mothers to help improve the likelihood of giving birth to a healthy child, some of which include:

- Eating healthfully during pregnancy
- Avoiding the usual nasties like alcohol and tobacco
- Staying fit and active

But there are more than enough books, blogs, and magazines out there to help you to maintain a healthy lifestyle when it comes to eating and exercise during pregnancy, so that's not what I want to cover in this book.

Your labour and childbirth experience can be directly affected by your emotional and mental state and with adequate emotional and mental preparation, it is possible to achieve a natural birth without necessarily experiencing the pain that many assume comes with it. It's not guaranteed, but it's possible. And that was enough for me!

A lot of people, when they hear you're planning on having a home birth (which suggests a natural birth due to the limited options available for medical intervention), will say things like, "Ooh, you're brave!" or "Why? Aren't you near a hospital?" and assume that you're some hardcore hippy chick, which is ridiculous. Bravery has nothing to do with it. A home birth can be an amazingly enjoyable experience that leaves you buzzing and feeling utterly euphoric. At least that was my experience. For me, you have to be brave deciding to give birth in a hospital. The horrible environment, with doctors and nurses swarming everywhere, no privacy, increased risk of medicalisation, increased risk of picking up super-bugs . . . the list goes on!

In deciding to opt for a natural birth does not mean that I'm some freak of nature, a super fit yoga bunny or a hardcore hippie that feels no pain or lives in woo-woo land. I'm just someone who prefers the natural alternative when there is one, and who understands and respects the mind-body connection. Oh, and I can be pretty determined and focussed when I set my mind to it.

If you're curious about natural birth and are keen to understand why it might be a good option to consider, I've brought together the information that I used to help make my decision. What I'm sharing with you isn't the final word on the matter, and it's important for you to consider what is right for you. But I at least hope that this will be useful in thinking through your birth choices.

Why a Natural Birth Is Good for the Mother

Here are just some of the reasons why a natural birth is good for the mother.

Labour is usually quicker

Epidurals and other pain relieving medications often slow down labour, which means it may last longer. Pain medications can interfere with the body's natural ability to progress labour, which can slow down contractions. Also, as you tend not to feel the contractions (not always!), then you might not instinctively know when to push. By losing touch with your body in this way, it may mean that you struggle to work with your body in delivering Baby; this can mean not pushing at the right time, or not using the contraction adequately to push the baby out. Accepting pain medication might be a double-edged sword. On the one hand it can help to relieve some of the pain you're experiencing, but due to the effect the meds have on your hormones, you may start losing the buzzy feel of your endorphins. Some women say that labour stopped being enjoyable when their pain meds kicked in, even though the pain subsided. So, if you do resort to asking for pain relief, it's no big deal, it simply means that you're choosing a different birthing experience.

My first birth lasted six hours from the first contraction and my second lasted three hours. Many women have much faster births than this, and I was super grateful not to be in labour for hours and hours, if not days! I don't know whether my short birthing times were down to the preparation work I had done, but when you consider that average first-time labours exceed thirteen hours*, I like to think that it did.

*For a first baby, the average length of the first stage of labour is twelve to fourteen hours, the second stage is one to two hours, and the third stage is five to sixty minutes. For subsequent babies, women can expect the first stage to last around six to eight hours and the second stage to last from five to sixty minutes[17].

You avoid the potential avalanche of interventions

Choosing to accept drugs into your body can start well before labour. If you're past your due date, you might be offered a number of medical interventions to *get things going* and induce labour. The thing is, once a birth has been artificially induced, the normal physiology of birth has been disrupted and the body is unlikely to progress through labour as smoothly as it would have if allowed to progress on its own timetable. Interfering with the natural birthing process can cause a number of negative outcomes, including impeding the body's ability to produce its own birth hormones, creating opportunities for infection, exposing the baby to synthetic medications, and raising the likelihood of delivery by C-section.

Despite mounting evidence to the contrary, there is a disturbing trend[18] toward the overuse of birth interventions in the United States. The overall cesarean delivery rate in the United States has increased by 60% between 1996 and 2009, from 20.7% to 32.9%. The World Health Organization recommends that the C-section rate should not be higher than 5–10% of births.

Of course, this is not to say that once you've kicked off with a sweep or some other intervention you won't be able to continue naturally, it simply means that you've reduced the likelihood and have potentially introduced some risk into your birth. However, if there is a medical need for induction wherein the risk of doing nothing outweighs the risks of induction, then it's a no-brainer. But I urge you to not feel pressured into this decision, as it's not one to be taken lightly. According to research carried out by the World Health Organization in 2010, between 4 and 6 million C-sections are performed every year that are considered to be medically unjustified[19].

Faster recovery time

If you haven't chosen to be given sensation-numbing drugs, you'll be free to get up and move about soon after labour. If you want, you can get up, walk around, have a shower, and get dressed. After my birth I popped upstairs to take a shower so that I could settle down for a cup of tea and toast in my lounge with my new little one. It was a wonderful moment!

Euphoric or orgasmic birth anyone?

Women who have natural births often feel pretty amazing soon after giving birth, with some even claiming to feel euphoric during the birthing process, which then stays with them for a while afterwards. The euphoric feeling that many naturally birthing mums experience is caused by the release of endorphins in the body during labour. Endorphins are the calming and pain-relieving hormones the body naturally produces when dealing with pain, and tests have shown that a woman's body won't release nearly as many if pain medication is used.

When I was training in Laughter Yoga during my last pregnancy, I read that Laughter Yoga can help you to have an orgasmic birth. I was a bit sceptical to say the least, but I thought, "Hey! That would be cool," while deep down thinking, "If I can just keep the pain at bay that'll be OK with me." I mentioned this to the other women in the course and one of them, Rose, claimed to have had an orgasmic birth. Nobody there could believe it! Rose went on to tell us that she had her four sisters and her mum present at her home birth, and the usual joyful family banter was happening throughout her labour. From what she said, it sounded like they were having a right laugh! Well, all that laughing pumped her body full of endorphins adding to the normal mega dose that childbirth gives you, and it seemed to have tipped her onto a whole new level of euphoria. She said it was one of the most orgasmic things she had EVER experienced. While I can't claim to have had an orgasmic birth, I certainly experienced the euphoric high. I felt so high and buzzy after my second birth. It was pretty awesome.

Greater connection to the birthing experience

When you're not on drugs, you're able to stay much more alert and present to what you're going through. This enables you to be more conscious and connected to the experience of giving birth. Pain medications are there to numb your physical senses, but they do more than that; they can dull your other senses too. This might mean that you feel quite detached from the birthing process, like it's happening *to you,* rather than you being part of it, if that makes sense. Having read a ton of blog posts on this, the one thing that seems to be consistent among women who accept medical interventions is that many of them feel a bit rubbish about their birthing experience. Some women say that they stopped enjoying their birth the minute the drugs kicked in. By not feeling alert when Baby arrives, they feel they miss out somehow on those crucial first magical moments. It's worth bearing this in mind when choosing to accept medical interventions.

You feel invincible!

In my opinion, the word "empowered" is slightly over-used when it comes to women stuff, but this is one place where I feel it's entirely justified. Many women who experience a natural birth report feeling empowered. It's that sense of, "I can do ANYTHING!" - feeling invincible, powerful, and that you can take on anything. These feelings contribute to an overall sense of confidence. Being able to birth naturally and successfully making it through the extreme physical and emotional demands of labour often makes a woman feel stronger and less fearful about handling other challenges in life. Many women cite childbirth as being one their life achievements. That's a big friggin' deal! This is what's waiting for you on the other side: your biggest life achievement!

Freedom to move during labour

When birth begins with an induction, many hospitals require you to stay in bed during your labour and delivery. This is so they can monitor you and baby, and continue to give you medication intravenously. The problem with being in bed is that you're pretty much in the worse position for labour. By lying down you're not tapping into the force of gravity in helping Baby to come out; instead, gravity is encouraging baby to put weight on your lower back. (Ouch! Just a little bit painful.) Lying on your back restricts the pelvic outlet by up to 30%, putting unnecessary stress on the perineum and sometimes causing drops in foetal heart rate and other forms of foetal distress. Lying on your back can also play into any fears you may have around feeling vulnerable or not being in control.

Contrast this against when you have the freedom to move: you can walk about, have a shower, bounce on a birthing ball, hop into a birthing pool, or get yourself into any position that helps you to feel comfortable. You might still choose to lie on your back, but the key distinction here is "choose." If lying on your back is what feels right for you, then do it. But for many women it's not, so it shouldn't be forced upon them.

You avoid the drug side effects

Pain medication can be pretty horrid; after all, it's powerful stuff. And that means it comes with some unpleasant side effects. Things like nausea, vomiting, and dizziness could affect you during labour, while afterwards you might get a post-epidural headache, as well as the grogginess that comes from waiting for the drugs to wear off. And let's not forget that as the drugs are essentially numbing the bottom half of your body, you'll pretty much lose full sensation and this might mean needing a catheter. Eurgh!

Why Your Baby Wants a Natural Birth

It can be all too easy to get carried away with the mother's perspective, which is not a bad thing. But there's someone else involved here too. Someone who doesn't have a voice and the ability to speak up: your baby. So in weighing our choices, it's important to take a moment to consider what your baby might want, don't you think?

I chose to aim for a natural childbirth because I wanted what was best for my baby. When I was pregnant, I was conscious of trying to do the right thing for my baby, by doing things like eating well and avoiding certain foods and drinks. So for me it seemed like a natural thing to want to continue trying to do the best thing for Baby through my birth choices. Once I started learning about the impact of the various options, it didn't take long to decide that aiming for a natural birth was the right thing for me AND my baby.

Now, I say "aiming" because that's all you can really do. You never know how things are going to unfold on the Big Day. Any number of complications may arise, and your idea of a natural birth might have to go out the window. But I think it's crucial to understand our choices fully so that we can make better decisions, and more importantly, decisions that we can live with.

Better connection with parents

During a natural birth, the baby benefits from the abundance of hormones flooding Mum's body, which helps to foster a strong connection between Mum and Baby. Also, because they're more alert, they can use their instincts better. When an alert and active (undrugged) baby is placed on the abdomen of an alert and undrugged mother, amazing things happen: the baby and mother are able to create a strong bond. Because they are both flowing with oxytocin, the bond is a real chemical one that feels very strong. As the baby is alert, they are able to make significant and deliberate eye contact with the mother and her partner and respond to them. Some mothers who had difficult, medicalised births often say that it took them weeks to start loving their baby, as they missed out on that initial "love hit" that comes from having all the hormones flowing uninterrupted.

Easier to breastfeed

Baby will be much better able to find the breast and begin feeding through breast crawling. This simply does not happen when the mother and child are drugged, and as a result breastfeeding starts off on a much rockier road and Mum might find it hard to feel the connection with her baby. Difficulties with breastfeeding can cause Mum and Baby quite a lot of stress in those first few weeks. And, of course, it means that baby might be missing out on enjoying the goodness of their mother's milk.

Drug-free baby

I keep mentioning the side effects of drugs, but let's back-track a bit here. Why should a baby be on drugs anyway? Especially if they're not ill. He or she didn't choose to take them. A lot of mums spend their entire pregnancy avoiding certain foods and abstaining from alcohol (and recreational drugs, hopefully) for the benefit of the baby, and yet all that goes out the window on the Big Day.

When a woman has an epidural to kill the pain, essentially the bottom half of her body is numbed. But let's just imagine what it must be doing to the baby. Babies typically weigh less than 5% of their mother's weight, so it doesn't take Einstein to figure out that they must feel completely zapped; no wonder it takes them days to recover.

If there is a medical reason, that is a different situation altogether, but often medication (to induce or for pain relief) is dished out without there being a medical need for it. Sadly, the chain of events that lead to Mum wanting pain relief typically start with the mother being under pressure to induce. So if we really want to do the best thing for our baby, it's worth taking the time to be fully informed and confident about a decision to agree to being induced.

Less risk of a premature baby

Babies born naturally will arrive when they're ready, whereas if labour is induced, there is no real way of knowing if the baby is actually ready. Due to known inaccuracies related to the common method for calculating dates (see Chapter 6), there is a chance that the due date has been miscalculated, which might mean that it's too early for baby to come out. When a baby is pried out early it could be at risk of respiratory problems as a result of under-developed lungs and other complications from prematurity. The only way to know if Mother and Baby are ready is to let labour begin naturally.

Lower risk of respiratory problems

Babies born by vaginal birth have a considerably lower risk of respiratory problems. The compression of the baby's thorax expels the amniotic fluid during the birth process and helps to prepare the lungs to breathe air. There is an increased risk of respiratory distress syndrome and asthma in babies born by C-section.[20]

Babies may benefit from receiving protective bacteria

Babies born vaginally are said to receive protective bacteria as they pass through the birth canal. These bacteria colonise in the intestine and are crucial for developing a balanced immune system, from childhood right through to adulthood.

This has been explored by Toni Harman and Alex Wakeford in their documentary *Microbirth* and book *The Microbiome Effect*. This whole area is the subject of quite a lot of research at the moment as the search for evidence-based recommendations continues. I interviewed Toni on my podcast about this and it's a fascinating conversion.

Babies cope better

The endorphins (nature's "feel-good" hormones) that are secreted during an unmedicated childbirth have been found in the placenta and umbilical cord. These hormones may help the baby to adjust to life outside the womb, as well as make the birth passage more comfortable for Baby. Also, the process of labour is reported to enable babies born vaginally to cope with stress better than those born dramatically by C-section. Cesarean birth triggers a dramatic stress response that could set up a child to always over-respond to stress.

Less chance of developing diabetes

A European study in 2008 found that babies born vaginally had a **20% lower risk of developing type 1 diabetes** than babies born surgically.

Avoids the potential health risks associated with Cesarean delivery

Given what we know about the cascade of interventions, when the natural process of birth is interrupted medically, each intervention is likely to lead to more. If this continues, then the ultimate destination here is a cesarean. Cesareans have been associated with a significant increased rate of asthma and allergic rhinitis, and children born by c-section are also significantly more likely to suffer from celiac disease and to be hospitalised for gastroenteritis.

What Every Pregnant Woman Needs to Know

Now, I mention natural birth as being a possible goal, but the really important thing is to achieve a *positive birthing experience* for the mother and her baby, and that doesn't have to be a natural birth. It's perfectly possible to have a traumatic natural birth, just as it's possible to have a magical and gentle C-section.

It's important to consider the wider factors that can help you to have a safe and healthy birth, because at the end of the day, for most people that is what really matters. Some might argue that I'm being ridiculously demanding wanting a birth that was not only safe and healthy, but also improved my chances of long-term emotional well-being for me and my baby. So, let's just focus on the safety and health aspects for a moment.

Nurse and childbirth expert Judith Lothian, PhD, reviewed evidence-based maternity care practices and highlighted[21] those that increase the safety for both Mother and Baby. In her research, she reminds us that even though science and technology have brought us significant benefits in managing our health, current maternity systems are now even more riskier and that standard maternity care does not always reflect evidence-based care. Frighteningly maternity care for many women still appears to be "just as we've always done". This is why we need to do our homework and get savvy.

Lothian also refers to a recent report published by the Milbank Memorial Fund, *Evidence-Based Maternity Care: What It Is and What It Can Achieve*[22], which highlights two key things. The first point she makes is that we know what makes birth safe for mothers and babies, but that unfortunately the maternity care that women receive rarely takes any of this into account. And her second point leads on from this and it's that because evidence-based care rarely makes it into standard maternity care, birth is actually less safe than it should be, and in some cases, it's actually causing harm. The frustrating aspect of all this is that it could be avoided. One of the things that she says, which I love, is this: *"maternity care that "expects trouble" actually creates trouble"*. She's reiterating something we know already and that's interfering in the natural, physiological process of birth when there is no pressing medical reason to just increases the risks facing mother and baby. The important point in this report[22] is that those things that are best for mother and baby, isn't always what's best for the hospitals and maternity staff.

As such, she identified six things that pregnant women need to know in order to have a safe and healthy birth. I'm going to share these briefly here; however, if you're interested in reading her research in full (which I encourage you to do) then just head to www.ncbi.nlm.nih.-gov/pmc/articles/PMC2730905/

1. Let labour begin on its own

If we want to know if the baby is ready to be born, the answer is simple: let labour begin on its own. During those last few weeks of pregnancy, the mother's body and her baby are diligently preparing for birth. Mother nature is pretty fantastic, and for us to naively assume that "man" knows best is surely meddling where meddling is not required.

2. Move about during labour

When a woman is active during labour, the movements she undertakes have several worthwhile purposes. Not only do they help her to cope with her contractions, they help the baby to ease down the birth canal. The better the woman is able to cope with contractions, the more oxytocin is released, which keeps labour moving. Good so far, but that's not all! There is also research to support the idea that moving about and changing positions helps to reduce labour, helps to reduce pain, and leads to less perineal injuries and less blood loss[23]. So when you see women dancing around during labour, you know they're onto a good thing. Put that music on, get out your Swiss ball, and keep movin', Mama!

3. Bring a friend or doula for continuous support

What women need more than anything during labour is to feel loved, cared for, and encouraged, and to be surrounded by people that they trust. This helps keep oxygen levels nice and high, which is good for labour. For many women, this means being supported by friends and family who can help her to stay in her birthing bubble and free of needless distractions. This is especially important in the hospital environment where you're pretty much in public place.

Another option is to have a doula. A doula is a professional birthing companion who is knowledgeable about labour and birth and who can help to provide essential emotional support and guidance during labour. They are not medically trained, but instead are there to support the family. I've interviewed many doulas on my podcast, so if you'd like to hear more about what a doula is, what they do, and how they can support you in the lead-up to your birth, head over here.

Some women prefer to hire their own private midwife for their pregnancy. This can help to provide them with the continuity of care that we know is so important for mothers. Midwives all over the world are under a lot of pressure, so they are not always able to ensure that you receive the continuity of care that is needed. Hiring your own private midwife helps to ensure you receive the care you need that will be conducive to a safe and healthy birth.

4. Avoid interventions that are not medically necessary

As I've touched on already - what is often best for hospitals and maternity staff is not always what is best for women and their babies - many hospitals routinely put women on an intravenous drip and hook them up with foetal monitoring equipment. This does not allow the women to move about freely. Furthermore, they tend to restrict the woman's ability to eat and drink, just in case she needs to have a general anaesthetic later. Of course, some of these practices might be worth considering if the medical need presents itself, but they should not be considered routine. And yet they are, despite evidence to the contrary.

The routine provision of other interventions, such as epidurals and the use of synthetic oxytocin, is also called into question. We know that their use interrupts the natural birthing process and so these really should only be considered when there is a medical need, but alas, as we've seen, they are not. Every intervention has unintended side effects, which need to be taken into consideration before accepting them. When interventions are used routinely and without a specific need, the natural pace and process of birth is interrupted which means that the woman is at risk from the cascade of interventions. This in turn exposes her and her baby to even more risks.

This is why it's so important to get savvy about the choices that you will face during your pregnancy and birth. Some things will be presented to you as routine, and you might think that they are and accept them without thinking. Be vigilant and do your homework so that you're happy with the choices you're making, because that's what they are; choices.

5. Avoid giving birth on the back, and follow the body's urges to push

Lying on your back is super bad for a host of reasons. For a start, it usually makes labour more painful! This reason is enough to never recommend it, but let me share some more reasons:

- When you're lying on your back, you're quite literally

pushing uphill. The birth canal curves upwards when you lie down, so you're going against gravity.

- Birthing on your back can make labour last longer because the body has to work much harder to eject the baby.
- Being on your back reduces the pelvic opening by up to 30% compared to other positions such as standing or squatting.
- Birthing in this position increases your risk of experiencing an assisted or medicalised birth.
- Laying on the back constricts blood vessels, meaning baby and mother won't receive the optimum levels of blood & oxygen.
- If the baby is in a non-optimal position (such as posterior), then the baby is less likely to shift into a better position while the mama is on her back.

The tragic irony is that lying on your back increases the need for the very interventions that the doctors and consultants want you in this position to check for. Now, don't get me wrong, sometimes it works for women and that's fine, but you should decide if it feels right for you and not feel obliged or forced into it.

The reasons I cite above are all physiological and body-related, and already it's pretty clear that this practice should be avoided. But what about the emotional impact of birthing on your back? The emotional aspect is rarely considered by care providers, and I believe that if they truly understood how the very thought of having to lie on your back during birth affected women in the lead-up to birth (even when they're not pregnant), then maybe they wouldn't be so quick to force women to do it. Lying on the back during birth is directly responsible for feeding so many fears that women have around birth. I know this because my clients are telling me. I'm always having to explain that it's not a necessary part of birth.

Fear of losing control

When you're heavily pregnant, lying down on your back is a night-mare for lots of reasons, but I'd say the main one is this: feeling a total loss of control. For those reading who aren't and who have never been pregnant, it might be hard for you to understand, so let me try to help you. Imagine you're in bed and a large St. Bernard dog has fallen asleep right across your body. Now try to move, get out of bed, turn over, sit up . . . NOPE! Not happening! You're stuck.

In my last month of pregnancy, to get out of bed, I needed to swing my legs sideways to get some momentum going in the hope that my back would get up in response. It's crazy-thinking that's based on assuming you have core strength to draw against (core strength that has disappeared now that you're pregnant!). So, as expected, this typi-cally failed and instead I'd have to call my partner to pull me up. When I was having ultrasound scans, it was the nurse that needed to pull me up off the bed.

Now imagine going through that, but you're in labour. Whole different story and a few thousand notches up the "I feel outta control" scale. There are other aspects to a fear of losing control, but if we focus on the very fact that the woman finds it difficult to move her own body, then this isn't a whimsical fear, but a very real experience for her. *Fear of losing control* is common among pregnant women and this prac-tice feeds it beautifully.

Vulnerability

Lying on your back with your legs in the air and having a bunch of strangers looking at your wootsy is *guaranteed* to make you feel vulner-able. Just the thought of it when you're not pregnant is bad enough, but when there's a St. Bernard lying on top of you weighing you down, it doesn't bear thinking about. Childbirth is already a vulnerable time for a woman, and what she needs more than anything is to feel safe, secure, and loved; this is what helps labour keep moving at a pace that's right for Mum and Baby. When she feels vulnerable and not in control, feelings of safety and security are out the window, and fears come rushing in; this is very bad news for labour!

Loss of respect

I don't need to labour (!) this point too much, as it's easy to understand how lying on your back with your legs akimbo and having strangers (including men) looking at your ladybits is going to make you feel. And *respected* isn't it. As I write this it strikes me how utterly absurd the myth of birthing on your back is. The emotional impact of laying on your back is bad enough given how important the emotional state of mind is when it comes to giving birth. But the fact that it also **makes labour longer, more painful, more difficult, more risky, and less healthy** all adds to up a ton of very good reasons why it should be avoided as much as possible.

6. Keep Mother and Baby together

It seems strange to have to highlight this point because for me it's so obvious, and yet around the world we still find that babies are separated from their mother in the minutes and hours that follow birth. The baby has been living safely inside their mother for nine months. They have only just made the journey earthside and they're still adjusting to their new environment. Isn't it obvious that the best thing for baby is to stay with its mother so that it can feel safe and secure? The mother's body is designed to support her baby through this important adjustment phase, and skin-to-skin contact is crucial.

Chapter Ten

Identifying Your Stresses & Fears

U p until now, I've been sharing some things with you that we could describe as childbirth education. But, just knowing this stuff doesn't always help to reduce your levels of stress and fear. Our intellectual department is not our emotional department, so we can't assume that being savvy about something means we're no longer scared of it. If your fear is *fear of the unknown,* well now that you know more, a lot of that fear should subside. But often there's more to it than that. So now we're going to change the pace and focus; we shift our attention onto **you**.

If I'm to help you to reduce your stress levels and clear your fears, it's going to be much easier if you actually know what stresses you out or what scares you. Just having a sense of being stressed or scared isn't enough; we need to get specific, and this means you're going to have to get specific. I can't do that for you, but I can help you with it.

The next part of this book is going to be a bit like having a session with me. When I'm with my clients, our first session is often just spent chatting about pregnancy and birth: how things are going for them, how they're feeling, what's stressing them out, what they're worried about. So I'd like this part of the book to be like that. It's obviously a bit hard what with me not actually being there with you, and then that minor thing of us not being able to have a two-way conversation. But please just park those silly limitations for now and let's do this anyway.

The time has come for us bring to the surface those things that might be stressing you out, the fears you may have around the birth, and any other life stuff that deserves attention. I'll start by sharing with you the things I come across most frequently from my clients and my podcast listeners. Me doing that is not intended to *add* to your stress and fear, but more to ask you to look inward and decide whether whatever it is I'm sharing is something for you too.

If self-reflection is a new thing for you, you might struggle with figuring out where to start, so doing this will help. Even if you're not new to self-reflection, there is still value in going through this kind of inward exploration. It provides you a moment to shine a light on various aspects of your life in order to understand them better and decide for yourself whether they merit the kind of attention you've been giving them. Often we get swept along through life and don't give ourselves enough time to stop and think about stuff so that we can decide whether "Yes. This is worth stressing about," or "No! What was I thinking? I'm OK with this." So that's what I want to help you with.

The best way to proceed will be for you to read through this once and start making some notes of things that come to mind. Maybe find yourself a nice notepad that you can dedicate to your pregnancy journey and birth preparation. You might have one already! If you do, give yourself a gold sticker. If you haven't got any gold stickers, now is the time to buy some. Believe me when I say this: gold stickers will save your butt more times that you can imagine once your poppet has arrived. Anyway, back to this.

Once you've done this, let things sink in for a few days. In reading this you'll be focussing your mind on some things that either you hadn't considered before, or things that are weighing you down emotionally and taking up too much headspace. Whichever it is, by shining a light on them we're giving your subconscious permission to mull over them and figure out where you stand. It's very likely that in the days that first follow reading this, new thoughts start to bubble to the surface. You might start gaining clarity on certain things and perhaps new questions might arise about others. You might get none of this and that's fine too. But just know this: stuff is happening beneath the surface! If new thoughts come to you, jot them down!

Once you've mulled things over, you might find it useful to come back and read these pages again, just to see where your thoughts and feelings are now and whether they've shifted. I think it's important to take a pause and slow down at this stage because it's good preparation for when it comes to doing the clearance work. It's like when you're planning a project - you wouldn't start implementing the project until you were super clear on everything that you needed to do as part of the project. Same applies here. Your clearance work is your project, but until you know what needs to be cleared, it's a bit hard to start the clearance work.

This is why you need a clearance to-do list! As you read through these pages and start to figure out what you feel you need to clear, write it down. This is the beginning of your clearance to-do list. Keep this list somewhere safe and accessible so you can add to it easily. I kept my clearance list on my phone because I knew I could add things to it whenever and wherever. But you choose what's right for you.

Over the next few pages, we're going to explore:

- Pregnancy stresses that get in the way of you enjoying your pregnancy
- Birth planning stresses that might be overwhelming you
- Life stresses that need attention
- Childbirth fears that you would rather do without
- Previous experiences that may have been traumatic or difficult that are affecting how you feel about your birth

OK. Are you ready?

Let's go!

Pregnancy Stresses

M y stresses had a life all of their own during my pregnancies. They would come and go, evolve, disappear and re-appear. New ones would show up, some would increase, others would disappear as quickly as they arrived. My hormones clearly didn't help, but given that it's a period of enormous change, on the inside and the outside, this is not entirely surprising.

Your Stresses Will Change

As you think about your stresses, bear in mind that you need to:

- Consider where you are in your pregnancy
- Remain self-aware and revisit them often so that you capture the new ones that have popped into your life, but also notice the ones that have slipped away

It's a time of huge change in your life, but we're adaptable beings. For some of us that means that once we get used to something, the stress it might have caused us initially starts to subside. But that might mean that new stresses jump right in to replace them.

I remember I had a bunch of pregnancy books that I would devour every night to find out what was happening to my body and to Baby. I would read blogs too, often re-reading stuff I'd already read, probably for reassurance that things were going well and that whatever was happening to me was "normal." All this was probably driven by my fear of having another miscarriage. The thing is, when you read so many books, articles, and blogs about pregnancy, you can't help but come across the things that could go wrong, especially online. There's nothing worse than coming across a list of the symptoms to look out for that mean you have to "seek medical attention immediately." Scary stuff, right? No wonder you get stressed by it all. I know I did. Any little thing I was experiencing that either wasn't on the list of 'things to expect" or was on the list of "see your doc ASAP" would freak me out and make me worry that this was yet another sign of a serious underlying issue.

The truth is that we're all so different and unique, our bodies will respond very differently from one another depending on all sorts of things - our health, age, weight, diet . . . our stress levels - and what might be a "normal' reaction for one woman might not be for another. And sure, don't get me wrong, there are times when we DO need to see a doctor or our midwife about what's happening to us. But for the most part, a lot of what we read is needless scaremongering that contributes to the low-level hum of stress that we need to steer well clear of.

In addition to working with a lot of pregnant women (myself included), I also receive a lot of emails from the women who do my online programmes telling me how they're feeling and what they're experiencing. This has enabled me to identify some of the most common things that tend to cause stress in pregnancy. Over time, I've noticed that stresses tend to be different depending on which trimester you're in. So, as I try to help you to identify your pregnancy stresses, I'm going to break it down by trimester.

First Trimester

PREGNANCY PANICS

Here are some of the common emotional hurdles you might come across during your first trimester.

OMG! I'm pregnant!

This is probably the first emotional bump in the road for you. It might be panic, shock, elation, or relief. The idea of being pregnant can take a bit of getting used to at first. But it probably won't be long until you reach the excited bit of "OMG! I'm going to have a baby!"

Even though the emotion you might be experiencing at this point might be positive, excess positive emotion can still put your body into a stressful state, especially if you can't sleep because of the excitement. Your heart might be racing, your breathing might speed up, and you might feel all tingly. Only consider working on this if the excitement of it all is having a negative affect on you or if you are feeling completely shocked and overwhelmed.

Having a miscarriage

Miscarriage is the loss of a pregnancy in the first twenty weeks. Anything from 10–20% of known pregnancies end in miscarriage, and more than 80% of these happen before twelve weeks. So it's a very real fear, particularly if you've already experienced a miscarriage. For some women this dominates their headspace in the first trimester, until they've reached the magic week number twelve when the risks decrease. There are so many unknowns when it comes to the causes of miscarriage that it can often feel like a hopeless lottery, but worrying about it constantly isn't going to help. Clearing this fear is worth doing if only to quiet the mind and reduce the physical effects of stress on the body.

Work & Career

There's no escaping it: pregnancy and kids are going to derail your work to some degree. Whether you're going to take the minimum maternity leave possible and head right back to your job full-time, work through your maternity leave with a newborn because you have your own business (like I did for my first - not easy!), or take a full year of maternity leave and go back to work part-time, your work is going be to affected. Not only that, but your long-term income-earning potential is quite likely to be affected, unless you're with a guy who's going to be a stay-at-home dad. These are very real worries that matter and have the potential to really impact your life.

In working on these, what we're not going to be able to do is to take these problems away, but we will at least reduce the negative impact they might be having on your headspace. Worrying or being stressed out about these things is not going to help you. Much better to remove the emotional energy around something so that you can fell calmer about it and think clearly so that you can find a solution or a workaround.

Relationship with partner

If this is your first pregnancy, then understandably you'll be wondering how this will affect your relationship with your partner. If you're in an established relationship in which a commitment has been made, then you'll be in very a different place from someone who's in a more casual relationship. Any worries you have about your relationship will need to be addressed and working on the emotional aspects of them will help you to remain calmer when the time comes for you to discuss them with your partner.

Sex life

Maintaining an active sex life might not be easy for you during your pregnancy, and might well become trickier as you near the end (although you might fancy a bit near your due date to bring on labour!). Having said that, you might also find that your sex life ramps up a notch. Sex post-children is different whichever way you look at it, namely because you just can't guarantee the privacy and freedom you used to enjoy, and you might be too knackered to even think about it, let alone do it, for a while. But add to that the changes that have happened to your body and how your birthing experience affects how you feel about yourself and you're sure to experience some kind of shift. That's not to say it will be a negative shift. Birth can be so magical too, and it's quite possible that your partner will be in complete awe of you and what you've achieved.

Telling others

For many, this will hardly be a source of stress, and will in fact be a huge delight and super exciting. But there still might be some stressful aspects to telling other people. Perhaps you have family members waiting in the wings who will inundate you with well-meaning or patronising advice. If you're married, these may well be the same family members who have been pestering you to have kids ever since you got back from your honeymoon.

You might have friends who are struggling to get pregnant or undergoing IVF treatment, or friends who have recently had miscarriages. This can be difficult for both of you. On the one hand you might be over the moon, and your friend may well share your happiness, but she will also be feeling a lot of pain and "why not me?" emotions. You may even find some friends will find it too painful to be around you, watching you grow, and so your friendship will become a bit more distant for a while, if not forever. I've had friends that stopped contacting me altogether when I became pregnant and I've never heard from them since.

If it's your first pregnancy, these experiences can be quite shocking or traumatic depending on the relationships involved. They also highlight the new life-step change that you're about to go through, which can feel scary. It's at times like this that you might experience a sense of loss or grief at the part of your life that you're going to leave behind. If this does happen to you, then it's important to face your feelings and figure out what it is that you're feeling. Even deeply negative feelings need to be embraced for you to move through them. Hidden within these feelings might well be the fear of motherhood as you emotionally hold on to the past and resist letting go, wherein you see motherhood as the start of a new life phase that seems totally overwhelming. If they're not cleared during your pregnancy, these fears can surface subconsciously during the birth and have negative effects.

Let's just say you have a fear of motherhood and what it represents because of what you'll be leaving behind; imagine how that might affect you during labour. On some level you might resist the birth as you hold on to what you have in life and this might lead to a long, slow labour.

Practical worries

Then there's all the practical stuff to worry about. Having a baby is life-changing, that's for sure. It can feel quite overwhelming with so many things to think about, especially if your pregnancy caught you by surprise and you realise that you have to move house. Suddenly there's a whole new level of stress piling on. You might start having worries relating to the home you're in, your car, your finances or perhaps child-proofing your living space.

Taking maternity leave

Taking time off work can be a wonderful break for many. I say "break," but it's hardly a holiday! Even if you decide to take a bit of time off before the birth, you're not exactly in the kind of state to do much. You can't really travel, not that you would want to, and even a trip into town can seem completely impossible.

If you're employed, the period leading up to your leave can build up to be quite a stress as you prepare handover notes, train new staff, and try to get as much done as you can before you leave. At this point you might relish the break you're about to have, but you might also be worrying about what job you'll be able to come back to. Will you want to do full-time work? If you want part-time work, will you employer have that available for you? Not knowing what you'll want, and therefore a general sense of not knowing, can be a little unsettling

If you run your own business or don't have paid maternity leave, the idea of maternity leave might be pure fiction. You might be able to take off a month but for you, it's very possible that you might be worried that you won't have enough time to spend with your baby.

Taking a break from our work can really help us to better understand how we feel about it. A lot of women use their maternity leave to think about changing direction in their lives. The arrival of a child can be a good reason to do this, especially if you think the full-time work you currently do is not very compatible with being a parent, such as juggling childcare and all the other disruptions that come with being a working parent.

Eating, nutrition, and being healthy

Now that you're pregnant, you won't be short on advice about the kind diet you should be following: healthy, nutritious, and balanced. If this is how you currently eat, then pregnancy will not be too challenging for you. Eating unhealthily when you're pregnant is not that brilliant for the baby, nor for you. You'll feel more sluggish and tired, and some of your pregnancy symptoms will feel more intense, especially things like heartburn. But I guess the most stressful aspect when it comes to food is that list of foods you're told you need to avoid. You can choose whether to follow this advice to the letter or ignore it, and if you're at home ignoring it then it's easier. But heaven help you if you decide to ignore the healthy eating and drinking advice while you're out and about! Other people will be more than happy to comment and judge you for it, so prepare for that. It can feel relentless to hear other people's comments and judgments, especially when some of what is said to you is based on questionable advice.

If this aspect becomes a sore point for you, it won't be long before you start snapping and biting people's heads off. It's best not to let it get out of hand, and to work out how you feel about these busybody comments and clear the stress around it. This is whether you choose to eat healthily or not . . . you will still get cheeky comments, so it depends on how you feel about receiving them.

Morning sickness

This can be a real challenge for some women, and can vary from feeling slightly nauseous to not being able to keep any food down whatsoever. I want to look at morning sickness individually because this is one pregnancy symptom in which there is an element of consistency as to what it may be linked with emotionally. So, if this is you, there may be hope.

You might be wondering what kind of emotional challenge could possibly be linked to morning sickness, and while I don't have the definitive answer, I would like to share something with you that might help as I know it's worked for many others.

Morning sickness can sometimes be a sign that you haven't fully connected with your baby and it can often affect women who have previously had a miscarriage. For some women, the loss they experience from going through a miscarriage forces them to detach emotionally from the little one growing inside. They don't want to become attached to their baby too much in case they lose them again. So they remain detached and disconnected from the life force that's growing within. A friend of mine who's had two miscarriages reported that she had awful morning sickness during her first trimester but that once she'd had her twelve-week scan and saw that her baby was OK, her morning sickness stopped. One of my podcast guests, Charan Surdhar, works on this a lot with women and talks about it during my podcast chat with her. You can listen to that here.

Frustration around feeling tired and exhausted

This was such a biggie for me in my second pregnancy. I didn't notice it in my first, though. My second pregnancy was just so exhausting that I could barely get home from work before I had to go to bed. On weekends I couldn't stay up for more than two hours before having to eat and then go and lie down. This total exhaustion really got me down, as I had to start putting an end to lots of things in my life including my business and one of my podcasts, not to mention household chores, playing with my daughter, doing family activities, and seeing friends. It all had to stop because I just couldn't do it.

But then I figured out what the problem was: it was me! Me, trying to do too much and not honour what my baby and my body needed. Once I accepted that this was what my pregnancy was like and that my baby needed this level of energy from me, I made this huge shift. I consciously stopped lots of things in my life that I had been trying and failing to do. And I embraced needing my bed (with a spare banana on my bedside table to give me the energy to get out of bed again).

I'm sharing that with you in case it resonates and helps. But I also realise that it's easy for me to sit here and say, "Oh! Just accept it honey!" when the truth is that doing that can feel pretty hard. But our pregnancy journeys are there to help us to prepare for our life as mothers, and I needed to learn to let go of things and put myself and my children first. I suppose I still need to remember to do that even now. The process of wrestling with something and then succeeding is an important one, and the ability to let go is going to serve you well both during birth and as a mother.

Second Trimester

COPING WITH BEING PREGNANT

When you hit your second trimester, you've probably gotten used to the idea of being pregnant, so that will be less of a worry for you. You've probably also had time to think through some of the practical things, and of course you've made it past the magical twelve weeks so your miscarriage worries might start to subside too. But there's probably a whole new set of worries heading your way. Things like:

Your body changing

You will now start noticing changes in your body. This can feel quite magical and awesome, but can also trigger a bout of worrying at the slightest new thing being experienced. For some women, the idea of their baby growing inside is an awe-inspiring feeling, but not everyone feels that way. Some women, especially those who might be tokophobic, have real difficulty coming to terms with a living thing growing inside them with some describing this as being a parasitic experience wherein the parasite takes over the host and takes all their energy. I myself had visions of *Aliens* and *X-Files* episodes when I thought about it. This was something I had to work on in order to overcome it, so if this is you, give yourself the time and space to articulate what this is for you so that you can work on it and clear it.

Other aspects of changes to your body can also present worries or challenges. Perhaps excessive weight gain, or the sense of becoming more fragile and less strong or sturdy. In my second pregnancy I felt very delicate and fragile and was extremely hesitant to do anything too physical because I just didn't think I could do it. This was a far cry from my normal expectations of myself, and I found this difference hard to handle for a while. Moving to a place of acceptance is key for many of these, but that's not always easy to do.

Pregnancy symptoms

There's no escaping it - you're bound to experience some level of pregnancy symptoms. If you're lucky they'll be quite light, but they can also be pretty hardcore and painful, which at times can feel relentless and frustrating. And given that you're restricted in terms of the medications you can take, often you've just got to put up with them until you come out the other end.

It may seem odd, the idea of clearing the emotional and mental stress of physical symptoms, but it's really not if you consider that your body is a holistic, interconnected system. Often, when we experience physical disease, it's because our body is alerting us to something we need to address in our lives. But we're not going to be able to be open to what our body is trying to tell us if we're stressed or annoyed by the very experience of the symptom. Once we can calm the mind in relation to the experience, we're more able to connect to our body and listen to what the issue might be, and we're better able to take the action that is needed.

During my second pregnancy, the symptoms I experienced were cranked up somewhat compared to my first pregnancy, both in terms of the intensity and the sheer number. I have to say, it wasn't entirely pleasant. Each time something new came up, I would begin by healing the emotional discomfort. Sometimes that alone would shift it, or at least reduce its intensity. In being less bothered by something, you notice it less.

One night at three a.m. I was still awake lying in pain, so I thought I'd Google my symptoms. I'd avoided Googling for a while as the stress of what you find online is often worse than the thing itself. Anyway, I did it and found that I had Pelvic Girdle Dysfunction (PGD) or Symphysis Pubis Dysfunction (SPD). Basically it's when your pelvic bone starts to shift open (readying itself for baby to pass through) and it's opened too much or unevenly.

Not only was walking total agony, but I could hear my pelvic bone click as I walked. Sure enough, Google said that I was stuck with it until baby arrived. Google said that I could do some physio, but that it wouldn't go away until after the birth. NIGHTMARE!

So I decided to work on clearing any emotions that were contributing to it, trying to be super quiet in case I awoke my other half. I spent twenty minutes or so doing some clearance work and then fell asleep. I proceeded to have the longest stretch of sleep I'd had since being pregnant - a full six hours! And when I got up, all my pain and the pelvic clicking was gone. I was amazed!

All the next day, I kept saying to my other half how amazing it was that I managed to clear it just by working on my emotions. He replied, "But that's what you do; you heal by clearing emotions, why are you so amazed that it's worked?" I'm always amazed by the results I get (this is why I love doing the work I do), and by the sheer awesomeness of the human body and its ability to heal and correct itself. The body heals best when you sleep; my body had healed itself and needed me to be asleep to do it.

If you're suffering from pregnancy symptoms, I urge you to address any emotional issues - how you feel about them - that may be linked to them at the first instance. At the very least, you will feel less stressed by them, and at the best you might even get rid of them. A great book that helped me heal my physical symptoms was *The Emotion Code* by Dr Bradley Nelson.

How others treat you when you're pregnant

While it can easy to talk about this in terms of your pregnancy, it's actually a much broader issue because it touches on how other people make you feel based on the way that they treat you. It comes to the forefront when we're pregnant because people tend to change how they treat you, or you suddenly are exposed to new things people do that might jar with you. So in considering this as a potential source of stress, I encourage you to broaden your scope and also think about how people treat you generally and whether any of it acts as a trigger for you emotionally. This is one that has a real potential to show up for you during childbirth, so it may be worth thinking about any worries you have about the people who may be present during your birth and how they might treat you.

Personally, I used to be quite annoyed when people used to constantly lift things for me early on in my pregnancy, as it would trigger my sense of being weak and unable to look after myself. This was all my own crap and actually they were being kind and considerate, but I was grateful for these experiences as they highlighted other aspects of myself that needed to be healed. Later on in my pregnancy I used to hate it when people I hardly knew would come and feel my bump as if it were public property. I still maintain that this isn't my crap, that they were overstepping the mark, or at least my personal space. Just as I wouldn't hug someone I'd just met, I don't think it's OK for people I don't really know to touch my body like that. Is that just me? In any case, these experiences highlight aspects of ourselves that may or may not need attention to help us reduce stress in our lives.

So if you find you're being triggered by the way people treat you, take a moment to reflect on what they're doing and why it might be triggering you.

Third Trimester

How you feel in your third trimester will depend on how the rest of your pregnancy has been going for you. If you've had a reasonably healthy pregnancy with minimal symptoms and you've found the whole thing easy-going, your third trimester may well be a continuation of how things have been. However, it might go the other way. If you've been in denial on some level about the upcoming birth, as your due date approaches, you might start feeling more unsettled and nervous.

If you've been struggling with severe symptoms and have had some health challenges, by the time you reach your third trimester, you might very well be feeling like your pregnancy is lasting forever and that you just wish it would stop. My first pregnancy was a breeze, yet my second felt like this thing that went on forever. I couldn't believe that I still had another three months to go and couldn't imagine putting up with this for that long.

Of course, everyone's pregnancy is different so I'd rather not sit here and tell you how yours is going to be, but it's possible that if you've been trying to park things in the back of your mind, it becomes more and more difficult as time goes on. You might successfully be able to continue doing this, but I urge you not to, because if you do, you run the risk of everything biting you on the bum during labour.

I get a lot of emails from women who tell me that they've been fine their whole pregnancy and now suddenly in their last month The Fear has hit them. This may be because now it's all seeming so real that the reality of their situation has struck them. Or perhaps they've been so busy with work that they've not had enough head space to think about the birth and now they have. Please don't let this happen to you. It's perfectly possible to clear your fears in a short amount of time, but it's all the other birth prep that takes time too.

Your birthing preferences

At this point you should start to give some thought to your birth plan or your birthing preferences. Coming up with your birthing preferences is where the homework and extensive research begins. As you approach your birthing experience, the one thing that will serve you well is being informed, particularly when it comes to:

- Inductions and being induced; the risks and reasons you might choose to be induced
- The risks associated with waiting until forty-two or forty-three weeks
- The effect of pain relief on you and your baby
- The risks of a Cesarean and when or why it's worth considering
- The benefits and risks associated with a natural birth
- The benefits and risks associated with choosing to birth in a hospital
- The benefits and risks of water births
- Breech babies; what it means for a vaginal birth and how to turn them
- Your birthing rights

This list isn't definitive and you should consider adding to it to address any personal circumstances, such as:

- Choosing a vaginal birth after a C-section (VBAC)
- Being older (over forty years old)
- Being overweight
- Being diabetic or having gestational diabetes
- Experiencing high blood pressure

If there's one piece of advice I'd like to offer at this stage, it's this: don't wing it and don't duck out of this. Your birthing experience is too important for both you and your baby's future well-being to just leave your birth to chance and hope for the best. If you don't do your homework and you need to make decisions during the birth, you want to be in a position in which you've already done your homework and you're comfortable with your decisions. Being informed and making a decision that you can live with will go a long way to help maximise the chances of a positive birthing experience and minimise the likelihood of experiencing difficult emotions about your birthing experience.

** SHORTCUT ALERT **

My *Fearless Mama Ship* membership site includes lots of articles, videos and prep downloads to help you prepare and plan for your birth including downloadable birth plan templates for you to tweak and make your own. Find out at www.fearfreechildbirth.com/join-fearless-mama-ship/

As you start to engage more fully in the practical aspects of your upcoming childbirth, it's possible that certain birthing options will be taken or rejected from a place of fear. For example, you might choose not to give birth at home because you're fearful of pain and want to have access to plenty of pain relief. Perhaps you have a fear of injections and so you decide to dismiss epidurals. Or maybe your fear of giving birth is leading you down the road to a C-section.

Whatever comes up as you work through your birthing preferences, make a note so these things can be worked on later. When I did this, I realised that I was choosing a highly medicalised birth (with a C-section as my plan B) because of my fear of pain. Once I'd cleared my fear of pain, I was no longer drawn to these choices and other options became available to me.

So now that we have the super important practical stuff out of the way, what other stresses might you be experiencing at this point? Here are a few that may resonate with you:

Baby's name

This is an interesting one! Perhaps you've decided that you're going to find out the sex of your baby and in fact you already have a name lined up. In which case, this is not even a thing for you. If you've got two names sorted out, it won't even be a thing for you if you've decided not to find out what sex your baby is.

But, if like me, you decided not to find out the sex of your baby and have no idea whatsoever on names, this might get a bit stressful. I remember buying books on names, reading lists of names from all over the world, anything to get inspired for the name of my child. Things were made all the more difficult because my other half and I could never agree on anything name-wise and it just felt like the whole name thing dragged on forever. Well, it did actually. Our first-born was finally given her name when she was ten days old - the latest possible time before we had to get her birth registered! Don't you love a bit of lastminute.com?

What really annoyed me about that whole episode were the friends and family pestering us all over social media and via text demanding to know the name so that they could send a card. During that phase almost daily I'd be shouting, "The baby can't read! You're sending the card to us, the parents!" at my laptop.

But if you have got a name figured out, that doesn't mean you're off the hook. These well-meaning friends and family are quite possibly going to jump in with opinions and judgements on whatever you've chosen. I recommend a similar strategy to the *How to Avoid Due Date Stress* strategy: say nothing or be the Queen of Vague and then surprise them *after* the event.

Stopping work

If you have a job or a business, it's unlikely that you'll be taking it easy in the final weeks of work. Instead, you might well be drowning in handover lists or trying to nail that ridiculous to-do list before you stop. I realise I can't do anything about your workload or your boss, but I would like to remind you that even though you might think this stuff matters, it doesn't. Not really. Six months down the line when you're enjoying your new little baby, will you be wondering about that to-do list that you never got to finish? Probably not. This is the time to start clawing back. This is the time to start claiming what you deserve and what you and your baby need. Practice now. You'll need to be well-versed in this during the birth and as a new mum. You and your baby need you to take it easy and not get needlessly stressed about to-do lists. Just let it go!

Getting everything ready for baby's arrival

Some people go crazy with this stuff. In fact, some people are so crazy that they have the whole nursery kitted out before they reach twelve weeks. Well, maybe they're not crazy, but I suppose they probably also have all their Christmas shopping done by February and in my head, this is crazy behaviour. As I've already mentioned, I'm more likely to be found turning up late at the lastminute.com school of thinking, so having the nursery ready months in advance would simply never feature in my reality.

In fact, during my first pregnancy we had a ton of major DIY work to get done in order for the nursery to be ready; think knocking down walls and bathroom installs and you might be close. I think the paint finally went down a week before my due date and at that point we still didn't have a cot. I'm pretty sure that all we had was the bare minimum: the car seat and a pram. To be honest, you don't even need a nursery for the first few weeks because Baby will probably be sleeping in the same room as you. So you can chill out about the state of your nursery if you're having a slight panic attack about what still needs to happen.

All you really need at the beginning is a Moses basket, nappies, bodysuits, and a huge pile of muslin cloths. Anything else is pure marketing BS. Don't get me wrong, as the weeks go by, you start to need new things, different things, which continues for about eighteen years until they leave home! And that's why we have Amazon and eBay apps on our mobiles: so that when you're awake doing another feed at three a.m. and realise something else that you think you need, you buy it and it arrives in the next twenty-four hours. Buy what you need when you need it, rather than anticipating you might need it. As someone who has my marketing BS radar on high alert (I used to work in marketing and I know all the tricks), I still got suckered into buying loads of crap I never used.

Your Childbirth Fears

I f you're to have a fearless childbirth, then this is where the magic happens. But in order for you to enjoy the calm waters of your positive birthing experience, we must first dive into the murky waters that are your fears. There's no way around this, I'm afraid. So put on your goggles and let's jump right in!

The simplest way to approach this task is to just start jotting down the things that scare you around birth. When I first did this, I had pages of things and it felt quite overwhelming. But the longer I sat with them, the more I realised that there was a lot of overlap and some key themes were emerging. You might find this too. But to start with, just write everything down and don't get too bogged down with wondering about themes.

Since I've been helping women with their fears, I've noticed that there are some fears that show up time and time again. They might not all be called the same thing, though. I had one lady who recently thanked me for labelling one of my fears as a fear of pain. She had never really thought of it like that but realised that it was her biggest fear too; she had always thought it was something else. So to start things off I'm going to share with you some of the most common fears that I come across. This is not to scare you into a blubbering mess, but instead to help you to find the language to describe what might be going on in your head or your heart.

As someone who had a ton of fears, and more importantly as someone who's cleared them, I know how overwhelming it can feel when your fears get the better of you, especially when you have quite a few on your plate. It can also be time consuming to figure it all out AND clear them. So to help make things easier for you I've created some Fearless Birthing Meditations. This means that all you have to do is sit back and listen to me, rather than craft your own fear clearance scripts. Of course, that's only if I've made a meditation for one of your fears. We're all different, so you will probably still need to address some fears that are unique to you, but at least these should help speed things up for you.

The full collection is available on my website at www.fearfreechildbirth.com/products/

Fear of childbirth

This is a great place to start when it comes to clearing your fears around birth. Well, to be honest, when it comes to anything: start at the broadest level and work your way down to become more specific as time goes on.

If you're tokophobic, you are definitely going to want to start here. It might well be that you're so fearful that you can't quite figure out what it is exactly that your fearful of, just the whole idea of childbirth.

Once you work on clearing your fear at this top level, it helps you to break down your fear to give you more clarity and understanding as what's happening beneath the surface. The idea of childbirth might be masking something else underneath. Perhaps you have fears when it comes to medical procedures or environments, or maybe you're squeamish and hate gory stuff with blood and body parts, or perhaps it's the idea that childbirth represents the gateway to motherhood and you have issues with letting go of your current life and embracing your next chapter. Any one of these could be feeding your fear of birth, but it might not be immediately apparent to you. So starting here helps you to break it down.

Once I'd cleared my overall fear of birth, it started becoming much clearer to me what my fears were, and many of them were those that I talk about below. Based on all the emails I get from women telling me their fears, I now know that they're actually pretty common. Looking back it's now nice to know that I wasn't some kind of a loony-tune fruitcake: a lot of women have these! You are not alone.

To help you on your fear-clearance journey, I'm providing you with my Fearless Birthing Meditation for this fear for free. You can find it in your online resources area.

Fear of pain

I've already gone into quite some length about pain during birth, so I hope you have a better understanding of pain when it comes to childbirth. However, understanding something in our heads (intellectually) doesn't always affect how we feel about it in our hearts (emotionally). It's very possible that even though you've read and understood how and why pain shows up in birth and that it's actually possible that it might not show up, you might still be thinking "Sure! But I'm still terrified of experiencing it!" After all, childbirth is hardly the kind of thing you go through without noticing any physical sensations. What will be important for you on the Big Day is how you choose to interpret and label those experiences. But we're far from that moment right now (as I can't imagine you're in labour reading this!), so let me just help you to think through how you might tackle your fear of pain.

The first thing is to make peace with the idea of pain, so that pain itself is no longer an emotional trigger for you. I would imagine it's more likely that you fear something you hate the thought of, whereas if you feel a bit "meh" about something, you're less likely to be fearful of it. Does that make sense?

So if you want to tackle your fear of pain, I encourage you first to simply think of working on the idea of pain, and then, if the thought of pain still freaks you out, to work on your fear of it.

** SHORT CUT **

If you want to save time, you can listen to my Fear of Pain Fearless Birthing Meditation which you can grab here www.fearfreechildbirth.-com/product/fear-of-pain/

Experiencing complications

This is a very real possibility for everyone, and while I don't want to stress you out, it's important to be prepared, both practically and emotionally. In practical terms, this means understanding the risks and benefits of the various options that you may be presented with. When I say emotionally, I mean letting go of any strong desires for things to go or not go a certain way, so that any change of direction on the Big Day doesn't add emotional stress to the situation. I'll be going into more detail about this later on as it's really important.

For now, I'd like you to think about what *complications* means to you.

- *I don't want to deviate from my birth plan.*
- *I might have to consider a C-section or medication and I want to avoid that at all costs.*
- *What if I have to consider medical interventions?*
- *I can't bear the thought of the doctors may have to use forceps or the ventouse.*
- *What if my baby gets distressed? What will happen then?*
- *I'm planning a home birth . . . what if I have to go into hospital?*
- *I want a hospital birth . . . What if I can't get there in time and have my baby at home?*

Birth Prep Work

Now is a good time to start getting some emotional insurance in place. Take your trusty notepad that you've been using to capture your fears and create a space for two columns. At the top of each column write the following headings;

1. My *preferred* birth will be like this . . .
2. My *least preferred* birth will be like this . . .

We'll be working with these two lists later on, so there *is* a point to doing this. No ducking out!

Fear of losing dignity

This is such a common fear among pregnant women. Well, not just pregnant women, I think everyone has this, but it's really brought to the forefront when you're pregnant because of the vulnerable nature of birth.

This fear can hold a lot within it, so if it's one of yours, it's worth giving it some thought to try and better understand what this fear means to you.

- *What will the midwives or doctors think?*
- *What will my partner think seeing me during labour?*
- *My partner will never be able to see me as a sexy, attractive woman after seeing me go through childbirth.*
- *The very idea of being exposed like that fills me with dread . . . all that sweating, screaming, and animal-like behaviour . . .*
- *What if my body evacuates my bowels during labour? The embarrassment!*

When writing down your fears, you might want to get quite specific by stating something like *strangers looking at my vagina,* or you might be OK staying quite broad in terms of *losing dignity.* It really depends on what's going on for you. If you find that all of these things are worrying you, then at least do the fear-clearance work at the broad level first before diving down into specifics. You might find that once you've done the broad level of clearance you don't need to do the specifics.

** SHORT CUT **

If this is one of your fears, I've created a Fearless Birthing Meditation to help you. You can grab it here www.fearfreechildbirth.com/product/fear-losing-dignity/

Fear of losing control

When it comes to control, there are different aspects that I think are worth exploring as the subtle distinctions between them are important.

HAVING control and BEING in control

Firstly there's the idea of having control or being in control; this typically applies to situations. Are you in control of what is happening externally? What people are doing, etc. If being in control is very important for you, then when other people have control instead of you, it can often cause problems, especially if you're a control freak!

FEELING out of control

This is different from NOT BEING in control. This is an emotion where you FEEL out of control, and it doesn't necessarily have a bearing on reality. We often hear people say how they felt completely out of control in a particular situation, and yet on the outside it looked like they had it together. So this is an emotional response. If this emotion really takes hold, it often leads to the next one, which is:

LOSING control

For many, this means emotionally losing control, losing a grip, not being able to keep it together. We can see this happening in someone when they might start getting emotional or angry. Or it could mean losing control of their senses or their body, like screaming or grunting. Someone who *feels* out of control doesn't necessarily become the person that loses it, though.

So when we think about birth and fear of losing control I think it's important for us to be really clear on what that means. If this is one of your fears then I'd like to invite you to give the following concerns some thought.

- Is it a fear of not being in control of how the birth is going?
- Is it a fear of losing it emotionally and crying, getting emotional in a way you can't control?
- Is it a fear of losing control of your body and pooing and weeing everywhere?
- Is it fear of losing control over the decisions being made about your birth? So the medical team *retains* control?

Having a better understanding of the various aspects of control can help us to figure out how to help you get past this. So if this is an issue for you, I urge you to give this some thought and take the time to work on this in advance of your childbirth.

This is a really key one to address if it's one of yours because a fear of losing control can only cause problems during birth. For starters, it's a fear, so will have a negative physiological impact on your body during labour and lead to things like a long labour or painful contractions.

Birth requires you to let go; let go of your need to be in control, let go of your need to control your body, let go of your need to control the situation.

THE ONLY THING you should be focussed on is staying in the birthing zone so that your body can just get on with it.

But it's not as simple as that. In fact, birth requires you to be able to play at both ends of the control spectrum simultaneously, at the BEING IN CONTROL END and at the LETTING GO END. You need to LET GO of your body fully; surrender all control to your body. It knows what it's doing. If this is your first birth, YOU don't; when I say *you*, I mean your mind, your ego (that's responsible for triggering the negative emotions). But your body, with thousands of years of evolution behind it DOES KNOW! Your body knows how to birth a baby.

But you also need to stay in control of your mind so that you're available to do what needs to be done. If you notice any painful twinges, you need to be alert and with-it enough to alert a midwife, or perhaps it's a sign for you to refocus your mind back on your breathing and your affirmations and less on your fears and inner chatter. So you need to let go of your body, but be in control of your mind AT THE SAME TIME, for hours!

** SHORT CUT **

If you'd prefer to bypass doing the clearance work yourself there is a Fearless Birthing Meditation available for this fear at www.fear-freechildbirth.com/product/fear-losing-control/

Your Baby's Fears

It might seem odd to think of your baby having any fears, and yet we know from a significant body of research that babies in utero are fully aware; they can hear, sense, and experience emotions just as we do.

Babies feel pain

The fact that babies feel pain is something that has only recently been fully accepted. For too long, scientists assumed that babies don't feel pain, although this was never based on science; it was always an assumption. This assumption led to many practices that seem pretty shocking once we accept that babies do indeed feel pain. Did you know that it has been a longstanding practice of surgeons to operate on infants without the use of painkillers[24]? Adding horror to this, it was discovered that major surgery on premature infants and children up to fifteen months of age was typically done with the aid of curare (Pavulon), which paralyses them but does not relieve pain. So while the children were experiencing the surgery fully, it was not possible for them to move or to even make a crying sound of alarm. Can you imagine?

Babies are alert to danger

We also know that babies are alert to potential danger when they are in the womb. In his book *Windows to the Womb,* Chamberlain shares a story about the baby of some family friends. When their baby's conceptional age was about sixteen weeks old, they attended an amniocentesis appointment. This is a medical procedure usually performed between nine and sixteen weeks gestational age wherein a sample of amniotic fluid is extracted from the sac for analysis. He writes, "She had taken her husband with her for this event, so with the ultrasound clinician and the doctor, there were four pairs of eyes on the ultrasound screen. The doctor had difficulty getting through to draw the fluid sample, but when he did, the hand of the fetus came up and batted the side of the needle."

This is not an isolated case, but something that is often noted among researchers. Other reactions have included the following: increase in heart rate, loss of beat-to-beat variations in the heartbeat four minutes after the puncture for two minutes, motionlessness for two minutes, significantly slower breathing for two days, and failure to normalise the breathing rate for four days[25].

While being viewed via ultrasound, a twenty-four-week foetus who was accidentally hit by a needle twisted its body away, located the needle with its arm, and repeatedly struck the needle barrel[26]! Similarly, in the midst of foetal surgery, an obstetrician reported that when he had a blood vessel all lined up and was ready to strike, a hand came out of nowhere and knocked the needle away[27].

These cases tell us quite clearly that babies in the womb have an understanding of things that will bring them pain, are alert to those experiences, and act accordingly, just as we would.

Baby's emotional awareness

When we consider that babies feel pain, cry, and are alert to danger, it follows that they experience emotions. A cry is an audible sign of an emotion. Just because we don't hear a sound doesn't mean emotions aren't present, but surely when sounds are present, isn't that proof that emotions are there too? For us to dismiss the idea that our babies do not have an emotional life in our wombs is simply naive. Much better to accept this and act accordingly.

Once we accept that our baby has an emotional awareness, it's not a big leap to consider that they might be fearful of being born. They know something is coming because they hear you and others talking about it all the time. If you've been sharing your own fears out loud, your baby will definitely think there's something worrying on the horizon. So, it's not surprising that some babies might prefer the idea of staying nice and snug inside Mummy's tummy rather than coming out into the harsh world and starting this thing called life. If you add to this Mum's stressed and fearful state and her belief that she can't birth her baby without help, then we have a perfect cocktail of birth resistance, with neither Mum nor Baby wanting to go through with the birthing process.

The thing with emotions is that they get trapped within our body, especially the deeply hidden ones or the big nasty ones. As part of our Fearless Birthing preparation, we're clearing the negative emotions from our mind and our body. But there is another little body and mind in there too that we mustn't forget, and it's hardly fair to clear our own fears and negative emotions and not clear our baby's too. So in the interest of being thorough, I believe it's important that we work on our baby's fears too.

If we don't, who knows what Baby might do to avoid experiencing the thing he or she is scared of? If poppet is scared of being born, then he or she may dilly-dally and withhold the onset of labour. We are still not clear what triggers labour. Some say it's when Baby is ready, some say it's when Baby feels as though there's no more room while others say it's Mum's body that triggers labour when the body feels it is approaching the end of its ability to sustain Baby healthfully. But wouldn't it be interesting to consider the idea that Baby will not be ready if Baby is scared. Just as you're not ready to jump off the highest diving board at the pool until you've overcome your fear of heights and deep water and gathered the emotional strength to jump.

How do we identify Baby's fears?

This is an opportunity for you to tap into your intuition as a mother. Take a moment to be still and connect to your baby. This might simply involve speaking to your baby in your mind and "listening" for a response. Whatever pops into your mind is likely to be your baby communicating with you. Be sure have a clear intention to "hear" your baby and not to project your own fears and thoughts. This is why it's important to learn to be still and to clear your mind. In taking the time to clear our own fears, we're creating the space in our minds for our baby to be able to communicate with us.

I've had many pregnant women share with me their stories of communicating with their baby, like Robyn, for example:

Silly though it may seem, I already spend time daily chatting with our unborn child and telling them how amazing our pregnancy and birth is going to be.

Sophie uses visualisation to help her prepare for her birth and communicate with her baby:

I used one of my visualisations to go to a lemon grove I often "visit," and my baby was waiting for me under a tree. I lay down with him and breastfed him, and told him his name and we had a long conversation. I told him all about his sister and his Dad and what those words meant, and tried to explain to him what the world is (a giant womb which we are both in and outside of) and what other creatures he will see and what wonderful things I have to show him. He then asked me about birth said he was worried about what he had to do, so I told him I would be there all the time and it was something we did together, that my body would guide him through my bone cave and then my flesh cave, and the first thing he would see would be my face and feel my hands holding him. He seemed much happier after that and when it was time to wake up, I left him sleeping peacefully nestled in the roots of a lemon tree.

If you're familiar with muscle-testing or dowsing, then this is something you can use by simply asking yes/no questions. You should start to gain a clearer picture of the thoughts and feelings your baby might be having.

This is what I used to help me to communicate with my babies before they arrived. For my first daughter, every day past her due date I would spend time with her, asking her whether there was anything that was keeping her from being born. Four days after her due date, I asked her about the name we had picked for her. She told me that she didn't like it. What followed was a tricky conversation with her dad to explain that we were going to have to ditch the name we'd spent hours choosing. She arrived the next day.

With my second daughter, I went through the same process. Each day I asked her if she had any fears or emotions that were keeping her inside and each day she would respond with a no. Until one day it was a yes. I eventually uncovered that she had a fear of being born (this was the day after my hospital meeting with the two consultants in which we discussed the risks of me being an older mum and her being stillborn and when we agreed I'd be monitored every two days). That day I spent a good hour clearing her fears around being born.

Chapter Eleven

CLEARING YOUR FEARS & STRESSES

How to Tackle Your Fears

Now that you've taken the time to identify your fears, a great next step is to come up with your fear-clearance plan. There are many ways that you can reduce your fears so having a plan is a good idea. We can't treat all fears in the same way, and what works for one person might not work for someone else. So I'd like to share some fear reduction strategies with you so that you an come up with a plan that suits you.

These two questions are a great place to start;

1. What type of fear are we dealing with?
2. How strong is the fear?

What type of fear are we dealing with?

In chapter one I talked about how there are two types of fears when it comes to pregnancy and birth fears, so I'm just going to recap them here for you along with some strategies you can use to address them.

1. Fear of the unknown

Fears of this nature are usually because you have a limited knowledge of pregnancy and the birthing process. If your knowledge of birth comes from magazines, newspaper headlines, movies and birthing reality shows then this is understandable. These sources are not trying to educate you about birth; they are vying for clicks, views and advertising dollars so you can't assume that you are being presented with well-balanced and researched information. Drama? Yes! Fear-mongering? Absolutely! Helpful education? Not really.

The good news is this; if your fears of birth are down to you not knowing enough about birthing, then you can easily overcome them by educating yourself about pregnancy and the birthing process. You might be tempted to watch some birthing reality TV shows. Please don't as this isn't considered to be birth education. Instead, seek out information that is intending to educate, or read some pregnancy and birth books, watch some pregnancy and birth documentaries and do research of your own. Taking a pro-active role in seeking out information about birth will help many of these fears slip away. But, if after doing this you're still fearful, then you probably have the next category of fears; deep-rooted fears.

2. Deep-rooted emotional fears

These kind of fears are unlikely to shift just by reading a pregnancy book. What makes these deep-rooted is that these fears probably have their roots in your subconscious and will be linked to things like your previous experiences, your beliefs or even your own birth. This means that to shift them we need a bit more than a shift of perspective and we'll need to go deeper. How you go about tackling these fear will depend on how strong these fears are for you and how much time you have left before the birth.

The first thing we need to do is determine how strong your fears are, because this will guide you towards a strategy that is more likely to help you.

How strong are your fears?
When we experience fear, there are varying levels of fear from feeling nervous or scared through being frightened up to being terri-

fied to the extent that the fear triggers panic attacks or leads to taking huge steps to avoid the thing we're fearful of. You can tell how strong your fear is by thinking about these questions;

1. What words do you use to describe your fear?

Strong, powerful words indicate a strong fear. Words like *terrified, petrified, scared* show a strong fear. Whereas mild fear might be described using words like *worry, concern, hate the thought of, can't bear thinking about* etc. Notice the language you're using when you think about pregnancy and birth.

2. What do you notice when you think about your fear?

Specifically what do you notice *in your body* when you tune into your fear? A strong fear will be felt strongly in your body. You might notice things like pressure in your chest, racing heart beat, sweaty palms, shortness of breath, tightness in your upper legs or arms, or you might feel hot. These are all sensations that might be triggered by you thinking about your fear. They will differ for everyone. If these feel intense in your body, then it's a sign that you have a strong fear.

When you put these two things together you should have a pretty good idea on the strength of your fear and this will help you to identify some ways of dealing with it. I would recommend giving your fear a rating out of ten. This will help you to decide how to best deal with it.

If you have mild fears (1-4)

These fears may well be the kind that we might file in the *fears of the unknown* from above. Mild fears can often be put to bed with some good education combined with listening to lots of positive birth stories. For some lucky peeps, this is all they need. It may be that doing this can go a long way to reduce if not eliminate your fear entirely.

Birth education
Positive birth stories

Birth education can feel quite overwhelming at first. There seems to be so much to get your head around because not only are you trying to understand what is happening to you, your body and your baby, but you need to figure out your position on the various pregnancy and birth choices you're facing. To help you prioritise, I would recommend learning about those aspects that relate directly to your fears. So if you have a fear of pain, then learn about pain. Learn about how the body supports you during birth. Learn about pain medication. If you have a fear of c-sections, learn about c-sections. Find out why they're important and what they involve. If tearing is a worry for you, then learn about it. Well. . . you get the picture!

While you're taking an active approach to feed yourself positive information about birth, it's also important to be mindful about the negative information about birth that you might be subjected to and to limit the bad stuff as much as you can. So avoid people who have a negative view on birth or horror stories that they love to share. If social media is a key source of information for you, then think about changing your feed settings; follow more people who share positive and inspiring information and limit your connections with those who spout negativity.

This level of work predominantly happens intellectually and at a conscious level. You are undergoing the process of *changing your mind* and this will take time depending on how much information you're consuming and the quality of that information and how quick you can change your mind. If you don't have much time left - like if you're in your last month - then using an emotional clearance technique (as below) will help you to achieve results quicker.

If you have moderate fears (5-7)

Moderate fears are best tackled with some focused clearance attention. Fears at this level might be bordering on deep-rooted fears which means we might need to bring about change at a subconscious level for the fear to clear. Here are two ways we can achieve emotional clearance for these kinds of fears;

Repeated positive messaging over a period of time.

Examples of this include affirmations, visualisation or hypno-birthing (hypnosis) tracks. For these to work effectively it is recommended that you use them over an extended period of time. This is so that your subconscious gets the message and changes. To have an idea of the time frame we're talking, then it might be useful to think about how long it takes us to change our habits or our default behaviours. Apparently it's 66 days[28]! Well, that's an average, the reality is that it sits somewhere between 18 days to 254 days for people to form a new habit[29]. And as we're talking about thinking and feeling habits, then this is a good guide. When we put these timings into the context of a pregnancy, it's easy to see how important it is to start this work as early as you can.

Emotional clearance technique.

There are some modern therapies that work very quickly at a subconscious level that you can use to clear any emotional blockages (such as fears). These can be used directly on any particular emotion that you may be experiencing and they can often do the clearance in one-go which means that you don't have to keep doing it. You can seek the help of a professional or do this work yourself. Some of these techniques also have DIY versions too which means you can do the clearance work yourself. I'll be sharing such a technique with you in a bit: the *Head Trash Clearance Method*.

To recap, these are some great strategies if you have moderate fears;

Positive Birth Affirmations
Visualisation
Hypnosis Tracks
Emotional Clearance Techniques

Combining the above with good birth education will bring you great results. The truth is this is a multi-pronged approach and if you use a combination of strategies, then you're sure to get the results you seek.

If you have strong fears or phobias (8-11+)*

Strong fears are probably best tackled with the support of a professional. That's not to say that you can't clear these fears yourself, but the DIY approach will not be for everyone. Some people prefer to feel supported in doing emotional clearance work and that's where a professional therapist or practitioner can help. If your fears and/or phobias are accompanied by high levels of anxiety or stress in other parts of your life, then I would urge you to seek the support of a professional.

If you have strong fears or phobia, then it might be best to hold back on the birth education at first because it might make things worse and not better. Depending on the severity of the fear or phobia, education around the subject of the fear could be traumatising. Some women with tokophobia are triggered by the site of a pregnant woman so undertaking birth education is going to be very difficult. I know that I found this very hard until I had cleared my fears. I couldn't look at the diagram of a birth canal without feeling a panic attack rising. My pregnancy books remained firmly shut for most of my pregnancy until I could handle the information that was contained within.

If you have strong fears, I would recommend that you start by working on the emotional aspects of the fear and only once the fear has subsided somewhat to follow-up with the educational approach once you feel able to.

* *I've put 11, because often, in my work with women on their tokophobia, when I ask them to rate their fears out of 10, they give me numbers way above 10!*

Birth Prep Work

I've created a bonus podcast episode that talks through all this and which includes a fear-clearance planner. To listen to this episode and to receive the fear-clearance planner visit www.fearfreechildbirth.com/tackle-fears-bonus-podcast/

Once you've listed out your fears, you're ready to make a start with your fear-clearance. I'm going to share an emotional clearance technique with you that you can use on all types of fears, whether they're mild or strong. Combining this with the other strategies I've mentioned such as education, positive affirmations and listening to positive birth stories, will prepare you brilliantly for a positive birth.

Are you ready?

How to Clear Your Fears & Stresses

This is where the clearance action begins and I share with you the **5 Step Head Trash Clearance Method**. You'll notice I start using the term "head trash" a bit more here. As I mentioned at the beginning of the book, for me "head trash" includes those negative thoughts, feelings, and emotions that we want to clear, things like your fears and stresses. But that's not all you can use this clearance technique for. I'll share more about this later so for now let's focus on your fears and stresses, and how you can clear them.

Step 1: Identify the head trash

Before you sit down to do some head trash clearance, you first need to be clear on what it is that you would like to work on. If you've read this book in order and followed my instructions in the last chapter, then you should already have a nice head trash clearance to-do list built up.

With this clearance technique, we work on one thing at a time, so pick the thing you're going to work on now and you're ready for step two.

Step 2: Tune in and rate it

This step is about connecting to your head trash so you can get a sense of how it affects your **mind** and your **body**.

When we're triggered emotionally, there are things we experience that tell us that we're having an emotional reaction. Perhaps we feel tight in the chest or sick in the pit of our stomach, or perhaps we get tense along our shoulders, or perhaps our breath speeds up or even stops! We might notice images or videos popping up in our mind as we imagine the worst possible outcome or replay scenarios, or we might hear voices - our own voice maybe - telling us what we should have done or judging what we DID do. There can be any number of things happening in your mind and or your body that let you know you're having an emotional reaction. Compare this to a non-emotional reaction wherein you're simply being, existing in a calm state and not really noticing anything that stands out, other than that you feel fine.

If we are to clear stuff, it's useful for us to become aware of how things affect us. The more frequently we take a moment to notice and observe, the more frequently we notice when we are actually being triggered. Since spending a lot of time clearing my own head trash, I can easily spot when I'm being triggered by something, which in turn leads me to asking myself what exactly it is that's just triggered me, and so the clearance journey continues.

So take some time to connect to how this is affecting your mind and body:

- Do you notice pressure or tension anywhere?
- How is your breathing?
- What do you notice in your mind?
- Are there any images or videos unfolding?
- Can you hear any sounds or voices in your head?

This is what I mean by tuning in. If you're tuning in to an extreme fear, I don't necessarily want you to completely relive it and freak yourself out. But you do need to emotionally connect to it. The more you're able to do this the better, so get as close to the true feeling as possible. If you've had a recent experience you can recall, then use that as a basis for how it affects you. Once you've tuned in to your head trash and you're connected to how it makes you feel in your mind and your body, I want you to consider how intense it all feels for you. For example, let's say you have a fear of needles. Now, if you were to imagine a nurse standing in front of you holding a needle, you might notice some or all of the following:

- Your arm tensing in anticipation of the needle
- Shallow breathing as your fear kicks in
- Racing heartbeat
- Sweaty palms
- Sick feeling in your stomach
- Tightness in your chest
- Emotion rising in your throat

When you think about ALL the things you're noticing, decide how intense all this feels for you and give yourself a rating out of ten. If you mark yourself ten, then it's super intense and pretty hardcore for you, whereas one or two is a bit of a non-event, and not really anything that bothers you.

In therapeutic circles, this is known as the subject's unit of distress (SUD), and is a useful measure of how much something is affecting you. It's helpful to rate yourself before you start so that you get a sense of where you're at in the beginning. This way, once you've done the clearance work, you can ask yourself again and see how far you've come. The businessperson in me likes this because I like measuring things and knowing whether they work. If I start at a nine and twenty minutes later I'm at a three, then I know I've had a pretty productive twenty minutes. Some people spend years in therapy and never shave off that much of their SUD.

I find it worthwhile to make notes as I go through my head trash clearance. This is useful for a few reasons:

- It forces you to stop and think. Putting thoughts into words has power.

- It helps you to stay focussed on the task at hand. Clearing head trash can be distracting - your mind might try to avoid doing this because you could be self-sabotaging on a deep level. Having a piece of paper in front of you helps you to stay on track.
- You capture your starting point. Clearing head trash can be powerful, and it can be all too easy to forget what you were like at the beginning. Seeing it written down in your own hand can be powerful as you later sit there asking yourself how it was possible that you ever thought like that.

I've created a *Head Trash Clearance Sheet* that I use to help me when I'm clearing head trash. It's a one-page PDF, and I print out a handful so I can get out a new sheet every time I sit down to do some clearance. You can find a copy of this Clearance Sheet inside your online resources area.

Once you've identified the nature of your head trash and given it a rating, you're ready to start the clearance.

Step 3: Get into position and clear it!

Clearing your head trash using the 5 Step Head Trash Clearance Method requires you to be doing three things simultaneously:

1. You need to be *thinking* of the head trash you want to work on.
2. Your hands need to be in a certain position on your head (applying pressure to known acupressure points).
3. You will be working through a psychological framework, in this case the *head trash clearance mantras*.

Let me explain each of these to you so that you're super clear.

Think of your head trash

Your mind needs to be *thinking* of the thing you're working on. We're working with thought-energy, and if your thoughts are elsewhere then you might as well not bother. This is why it's important not to be doing anything else while you're clearing head trash. Driving, watching TV, or listening to music are all big no-no's! To get the best results, when you're thinking of your head trash, it's best if you tune in to it AND focus on those things you wrote down in the last step (tight chest, racing heart, shallow breathing, etc.).

Applying pressure onto acupressure points

The 5 Step Head Trash Clearance Method uses the hand position that Tapas Fleming developed for her technique, the Tapas Acupressure Technique (TAT) which is shown below. It helps if you close your eyes while you do this in order to stay focussed.

The TAT hand position

Take one hand and put your thumb and your ring finger onto the bridge of your nose where your eyebrows meet, or where your glasses would rest

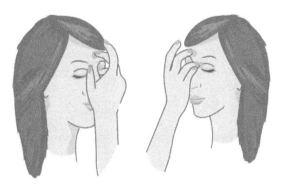

Using the same hand, place your middle finger in the centre of your forehead. This spot is often referred to as the location of your third eye.

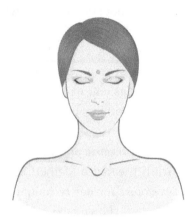

Place your other hand around the back of your head where the base of your skull meets your neck near the hairline so that your hand is cupping the lower part of your head.

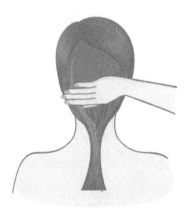

Switch hands to figure out which position you find most comfortable, but don't worry too much because you can switch hands during the clearance.

Raise your hands into the TAT position every time you say a mantra to yourself. You might then want to take a pause, at which point you can release your hands. Go back into the TAT position when you move on to the next mantra.

Work through the head trash clearance mantras in your mind

There are ten head trash clearance mantras in all and each mantra has a place in which you insert your own personal head trash. Until you become familiar with the mantras, it's probably worth writing them out in advance since you might need to tweak the sentence to ensure it still makes sense once your head trash has been inserted. This way you'll only have to read them out to yourself, rather than create them as you go.

You should repeat each mantra to yourself for about two minutes, or until you feel calm or done. You can say them out loud or just in your mind - it's entirely up to you.

The Ten Head Trash Clearance Mantras

_____ is a wonderful thing.

_____ is a terrible thing.

I love _____.

I hate _____.

I love other people _____ [being/doing/experiencing the head trash].

I hate and despise other people _____ [being/doing/experiencing the head trash].

I love making other people _____ [experience the head trash].

I hate making other people _____ [experience the head trash].

I love other people (or events and things) making me _____ [experience the head trash].

I hate other people (or events and things) making me _____ [experience the head trash].

Here is an example of the head trash clearance mantras, using frustration as an example of the head trash.

Frustration and being frustrated is a wonderful thing.

Frustration and being frustrated is a terrible thing.

I love frustration and being frustrated .

I hate frustration and being frustrated .

I love other people's frustration and them being frustrated .

I hate other people being frustrated (or experiencing frustration).

I love making other people frustrated (or experience frustration).

I hate making other people frustrated (or experience frustration).

I love other people (or events and things) making me frustrated (or experience frustration).

I hate other people (or events and things) making me
frustrated (or experience frustration).

Here is an example of the head trash clearance mantras using fear of needles as an example of the head trash.

Having a fear of needles is a wonderful thing.

Having a fear of needles is a terrible thing.

I love having a fear of needles.

I hate having a fear of needles.

I love other people having a fear of needles.

I hate other people having a fear of needles.

I love making other people have a fear of needles.

I hate making other people have a fear of needles.

I love other people (or events and things) making me
have a fear of needles.

I hate other people (or events and things) making me
have a fear of needles.

Practically speaking, this is how everything comes together: tune in to your head trash (while focusing on how it makes you feel in your body), raise your hands into the TAT position, and work through the mantras.

You might want to take a pause in between each pair of mantras to process the thoughts or feelings that have come up for you. If you do, then lower your hands from the TAT position.

Step 4: Rate it. Review it.

Once you've done the clearance work and been through all of the mantras, you're ready to check in to see how you've done. So, just as we did in Step 2, now we're connecting back to the thing we were just working on to see what we notice in our mind and body now. As before, you need to ask yourself questions like:

- What am I feeling in my body? Do I notice pressure or tension anywhere?
- How is my breathing? Fast or slow?
- What do I notice in my mind? Videos? Images?
- Can I hear any sounds or voices in my head?

And again, when you consider what you're noticing and experiencing, ask yourself how intense it all feels on a scale of one to ten. Remember, ten is super intense and zero is nothing. I'm hoping that you'll notice a drop in your SUD number. Be sure to rate yourself on EXACTLY the same thing you were measuring yourself on before. For example, if you're working on your anxiety that is associated with your fear of birth, then make sure that when you check in that you're measuring your level of anxiety and not how fearful of birth you are. Your fear of birth is a separate item on your list and not the one you have just worked on (anxiety).

Step 5: Clear the opposite

It is now time to do the clearance work on the opposite of your head trash. A great question to ask at this point is this:

What would I be experiencing if I didn't have this in my life?

So, for example, if you've just worked on *frustration*, ask yourself what the opposite of feeling frustrated is for you. Feeling calm? Certain? Clear? Motivated? Similarly, if you've just worked on *pain*, perhaps now you need to work on *pleasure*. There isn't a right answer to this question; it's very personal.

Here are some more examples to show you what I mean:

- Being ignored -> being listened to, getting attention, being the focus of attention, being spoken to
- Rejection or being rejected -> being accepted, being invited
- Fear of pain -> fear of pleasure, acceptance of pain, loving pain, want or desire for pain
- Messiness and chaos (kids, other people, home environment, etc.) -> Being tidy, well organised, pristine, museum-like

Once you've identified the opposite of your head trash (Step 1) you need to go back to Step 2 and repeat the clearance process (Step 3) followed by Step 4.

Quick Recap

Step 1 – Identify the head trash you want to clear
Step 2 – Tune in and rate it
Step 3 – Clear it
Step 4 – Rate it and review it
Step 5 – Clear the opposite (*go back and repeat Steps 2, 3 and 4*)

It's quite likely that you have a ton of questions about what I've just shared with you. Things like:

- How do I word my head trash for the mantras?
- What does a head trash clearance list look like?
- Why am I saying LOVE and HATE?
- This isn't hypnosis, is it? I hope I'm not telling my mind to think this!
- What happens when I do clearance work?
- How long does it take to work?

- What if my score doesn't go down?

Don't worry, lovely ones! I've got you covered. I'll be addressing many of these questions in a bit. But for now I just want to share HOW you do the clearance work so that you can refer back to this chapter and have the info you want without all the explanations getting in the way.

I've created a handy two page PDF that you can save to your mobile device summarising the 5 steps. You can download this in the online book resources area.

Chapter Twelve

Difficult or Traumatic Experiences

If you've experienced a difficult or traumatic experience, it's very likely to be contributing to your fears about your upcoming birth. A traumatic event is an experience that causes physical, emotional, or psychological distress or harm. It is an event that is perceived and experienced as a threat to your safety or to the stability of your world.

There's trauma with a big "T" and trauma with a little "t" and I think it's worth exploring the difference. When we hear about traumas, we're probably hearing about those "big T" moments: things like losing a parent, surviving a crash, experiencing the horrors of war, being attacked or abused, or experiencing a natural disaster. But I would also like to acknowledge the other moments in our lives that can leave us feeling traumatised. It would be really hard for me to even begin to list those kind of moments because they can be so different for each individual. Just because one person finds something traumatic doesn't necessarily mean that another person will too. The truth is, we come into each moment in our lives from the moment before, and those moments are individually unique to each of us and everything that has come before us. So while it might seem that we're experiencing the same thing as someone else, we're not.

I know that talking about trauma isn't very positive or pleasant, but it's important. One of my key motivators for my clearance work during my pregnancy was that I wanted to avoid a traumatic birth and the possible consequences such as post-natal depression. On my own journey to better understand trauma I was curious as to WHAT made an experience traumatic and if there was anything I could do in advance to protect myself.

So in talking about trauma I'd like to share what I've learned and that's for two reasons. Firstly, it's to help you identify those experiences you've had that may be considered traumatic, or that could be having a negative emotional impact on your feelings around birth. This is purely for the purposes of providing you with clarity on what could stand in the way of a positive birth, and is not to add negative emotional weight to how you're feeling.

Secondly, I believe that in doing so can help us to take steps to avoid experiencing them in the first place. Understanding the conditions that enable an experience to be a traumatic one provides us with important clues as to how we may be able to protect ourselves from experiencing them. And that can only be a good thing.

As part of my therapy training, I've learned that there are four things that affect how we react to a situation and that determine whether it becomes traumatic for us:

1. Our emotional landscape at the time

This is about where we are emotionally. Are we in a good place? Are we feeling strong and resilient, or are we experiencing frequent bouts of anxiety and stress day in day out? Are we easily knocked off our perch, or does it take a lot to beat us down? If you're someone who is emotionally and mentally strong, then you will be able to withstand difficult experiences more easily and perhaps even take them in stride. Someone else, on the other hand, who isn't as emotionally strong might get completely overwhelmed and feel totally crushed.

We can go a long way to protect ourselves from experiencing trauma by strengthening our emotional resilience. This means becoming more emotionally aware and addressing our emotional issues, or as I like to say it: clearing our head trash!

2. The event itself

Of course we can't experience a trauma from an event without the event itself contributing in some way. But this will be affected by the other three factors. We can't do a lot about this. But one thing is clear, it's not the event itself that creates the trauma, it's how we respond to the event. And this is something we can have an effect on.

3. The inescapability of the event

If the person feels trapped as part of their experience, this will have an impact on how they react. So we can see how experiencing war, being attacked, or surviving a crash are affected by the very fact that a person can't escape what they're going through. This is what makes pregnancy and birth such vulnerable times for women as they are both inescapable experiences.

But the idea of feeling trapped goes much further than this and is not always as obvious as it may seem. We can feel trapped even if we're not physically trapped. There's the emotional feeling of being trapped versus the physical reality of being trapped. Just now I mentioned some situations wherein you would experience both the physical reality and the emotional feeling at the same time, together creating quite an emotionally intense experience.

So what do I mean by feeling emotionally trapped? Well, some people feel trapped in their jobs, their relationships, their hometowns, or some other life situation. It's very likely that they're not actually trapped, they simply feel that way. They could decide to leave their job, separate from their partner, move away, or take some other action to change their situation. But they don't, perhaps because of fear. This grey area of feeling trapped is what makes some situations traumatic for some, while others might look on wondering what the big deal is.

We can go a long way to reduce our feelings of being trapped if we address some of the fears that are keeping us trapped or how we feel about being trapped. This in turn can help to strengthen our emotional resilience so we're less likely to be traumatised.

4. The meaning given to an event.

The meaning we give to an event and how we subsequently interpret it has a huge impact. Let me share a story that illustrates this beautifully.

A woman in one of my Facebook groups came forward one day to share her "traumatic birth experience" (her words) and talk about how she wanted help and support. Other women came forward to ask her more about her situation in order to better understand how they could help. She explained that she had just had her fifth and final child. All her other births were hospital births, but for her last birth she wanted a home birth. In fact, she more than wanted it; she *desperately* wanted it. She had her heart set on it and she shared how she had imagined it was all going to be and how much she had been looking forward to it. On the day of the birth it transpired that she had to be taken to hospital. It was "nothing serious" and she went on to have a "lovely, natural" hospital birth (again, I share her exact words).

Understandably, some of the women in the Facebook group were confused, trying to understand the traumatic element. She explained that she never got her home birth, that she was "going to die without having had the home birth" she had dreamed of. Her little one was one month old when she shared this with us, but she was distraught and was reminded of this every time she looked at her baby.

In this story, it's not hard to see what's happened here. This mother put so much meaning and emotional investment into a particular outcome that when she didn't get it, she felt traumatised by it. Instead of experiencing the joys of a lovely birth and a new baby, she was experiencing grief and loss. If she had prepared differently emotionally and mentally for her childbirth, and given the birth different meaning, much of her difficult experience could be avoided.

I'm sharing this with you because there are some powerful lessons for us to take from this story:

- The need to respond with flexibly to what happens
- The importance of being able to let go of certain outcomes and expectations

- The need to think carefully about the meaning we lavish onto things in advance so that we don't set ourselves up for a fall
- The importance of being grateful for the things you *do* have and focussing less on what you *don't* have

These are important *life lessons*, not just things we can apply to our pregnancy and birthing experience.

What previous experiences could be clouding your feelings around birth?

What causes trauma for one person doesn't necessarily cause trauma for another. It very much depends on our sensibilities, our life experiences, and our emotional and mental state at the time. It therefore follows that any number of life situations could be traumatic. What I'm interested in here is those experiences that may be affecting your thoughts and feelings around giving birth and becoming a mother.

If you've given birth before and it was a particularly unpleasant experience, then this will likely have a negative impact on your thoughts and feelings on a future birth. However, the extent to which it affects you will depend on how you still feel about that experience. If you've managed to let go, move on, and create some emotional distance, then you will find it easier to feel positively about a future birthing experience. However, if it still feels raw and painful and makes you emotional just beginning to think about it, then it is likely to contribute to feelings of fear and anxiety around childbirth. Even if you've managed to let go and move on in your conscious mind, that doesn't mean you've done so in your subconscious mind. You may think you've moved on, but beneath the surface it might still be causing you stress and it might well rear its ugly head just when you least want it to: while you're giving birth!

Thankfully, it is possible to reduce the emotional impact of prior difficult or traumatic experiences and create the emotional distance required so that they no longer affect you in the same way, thereby freeing you up to enjoy positive experiences. If you're currently experiencing a significant level of fear and anxiety around childbirth, then it's worth giving some thought to the kind of experiences you may have previously had that could be contributing to this. This was true of my own anguish about childbirth, and I'll share more with you in a bit, as the experiences aren't always as clear-cut or obvious as one might assume.

But first let me share with you the kinds of experiences that may affect your thoughts and feelings about childbirth:

- Previous childbirth, whether yours or someone else's that you witnessed or heard about
- Gynaecological experiences; maybe you've had medical issues, surgery, or complications that make you're concerned or overly worried about anything that happens "down there"
- Sexual harassment or abuse
- Domestic violence

If you have had a difficult or traumatic experience that you need support with, I urge you to seek support from a professional because this book is not intended to help you with that.

Earlier I hinted at those things that were contributing to my own birthing fears, and, like I said, they were not entirely predictable.

My own birth

Yes, you read that right. The day I was born was a traumatic day for me. This is not something I was able to verify and check with my mum as she had died before I got the chance to sort out my irrational fear of childbirth. But as I was working through clearing my own difficult and traumatic experiences, I had a hunch that this might need clearance work, and it turned out that it did. I was surprised at first because I don't have any conscious recollection of my birth, as I'm sure most of us don't. So this might sound a little odd, given that I didn't have a conscious memory of my journey into this world, but there is still an emotional memory.

Our conscious mind tends to begin storing memories from about three or four years old; before then our memories are emotional. This means that if you experience an emotional situation and it stimulates your senses - sight, smell, sound, taste, touch - then you have an emotional imprint. This is why tastes, smells, sounds, etc. can be so powerful for us. These emotional memories reside in our bodies as well as our minds. Just because you can't recall something in your conscious mind, it doesn't mean that it's not currently affecting you. It just means that you DON'T KNOW it's affecting you.

When the time came for me to do the clearance work for this, I had a huge emotional release that came out of nowhere and which completely took me by surprise. But it was how I felt afterwards that was more interesting. Up until that point I had this horrible, heavy feeling in the pit of my stomach whenever I thought of birth. It was something that I could never really put my finger on because I could never find the words for it. But once I'd done this clearance work, the heavy feeling disappeared. I felt much lighter and clearer about birth. I still had some fears, but it suddenly felt less overwhelming and completely do-able in terms of overcoming them and giving birth. The sense of my fears being irrational and extreme went away. I felt like I could approach my birth preparation in a very practical way, and the remaining fears I had felt like I was just doing the final tidy-up, whereas before I still felt like there was this huge mountain to climb.

Looking back, I can't help but think that my own birth was the traumatic experience at the root cause of my childbirth fears, and that it was because of this that I was so easily traumatised by watching a video of a birth at school. I was in effect being *re-traumatised*. I know that my birth was a hospital birth, and this could even be responsible for my long-standing fear of needles and injections. Perhaps the way I had been treated by the medical team at my own birth, and the injections I would have received quite routinely, were responsible.

Since beginning to write this book and as a result of doing my *Fear Free Childbirth* podcast, I have been fortunate to speak with many birth professionals. One thing I've heard consistently is this: our own birth experience sets the tone for the childbirth experiences we will have. So if our own arrival into the world was difficult - from the perspective of you as a baby, not from your mother's perspective - then the memory of this still resides within you and needs to be healed so you no longer repeat the pattern. If your arrival was difficult for your mother and you have grown up hearing how difficult it was for her, then this is certainly something you will need to work on and you probably have additional work to do. If your mother told you how awful and painful your arrival was, you may well have the belief that childbirth is awful and painful, so in addition to the emotional memory, you also have work to do around your beliefs when it comes to childbirth and what's possible.

So whether or not you remember your birth, I urge you to work on it. Similarly, if your mother tells you that your arrival was fine - for her - then I still urge you to work on it. Just because her experience was great doesn't mean yours was. I've already mentioned some techniques that can help you, but when it comes to healing your own birth, there is another I'd like to share: Rebirthing Breathwork. Rebirthing Breathwork is another name for "conscious connected breathing," a technique that is known to help people to recall their own with experiences in vivid detail and in doing so heal themselves. I interviewed a Rebirthing Breathwork specialist, Catherine Holland, on my podcast; if this is something that you'd like to find out more about, you can listen to that here.

In addition to my own birth story, something else was affecting how I felt about birth:

My parent's separation and subsequent divorce

OK. I admit this seems a bit far-fetched to be related to childbirth, but hear me out. My mum had my brother when I had just turned four. It was also around this time that my parents were divorcing. As a result of my dad not being around, I would help my mum quite a bit with my brother, and I have clear memories of helping my mum change my brother's nappies (those terry cloth ones that needed safety pins!) and seeing her breastfeed him. Little did I realise that the idea that motherhood was a huge problem for me. In my mind, babies, changing nappies, and breastfeeding was equated with loss (the loss and absence of my dad) and rejection (my dad leaving) and was not something I was in a rush to repeat. When children are young, the logical, rational mind doesn't really feature into their decision-making; they simply feel it emotionally. Many children think they are to blame for their parents separating even if the facts of the situation have been explained. Emotionally speaking, the explanation does not matter.

Even though this isn't strictly childbirth-related, it's very much tied into motherhood, which being the immediate aftermath of childbirth, makes it very relevant. On some level I was fearful of motherhood since the last time I experienced motherhood things - nappies, breastfeeding, and babies - it was a painful experience of loss. All this affected me massively on an emotional level, despite it not really making an appearance in my conscious mind. It's only once I realised the link that I retrofitted the rational explanation. It was a real "aha" moment for me, and was responsible for me being able to contemplate the idea of having kids. Up until that point motherhood just didn't feature in my imagined future.

As you see, your previous traumatic experiences need not necessarily be obviously linked to birth, so it's worth exploring this with someone who can help you work through it.

Dealing With Difficult or Traumatic Experiences

I want to start by saying this very important thing:

If you have had any difficult or traumatic experiences that are still affecting you today, please seek the support of a professional. This book is not intended to replace the help that you can get from a trained professional.

However, having said that, there may be difficult experiences you've had that we can take the power out of so they don't feel so emotionally painful. When I think about my own collection of traumatic experiences - and I've had a fair few - there have been some I've been able to work on myself, whereas there are others with which I needed help and support. Some were simply too emotionally painful for me to navigate alone, so I needed someone else to hold my hand throughout the journey. Some were buried so deep that there's no way I could have worked on them alone because I didn't know what they were, what I was looking for, or that I even had a problem that needed addressing. But there have been others with which I've felt courageous enough to work on them alone. Only you can make this call, but if you're not sure, just get someone help you. Please don't go all gung-ho brave on me. It's not big and it's not clever!

Reducing the emotional impact of difficult experiences

It's possible to reduce the negative emotional impact of difficult experiences and you can do that to past experiences or for possible future experiences. The approach is the same. Do you remember when I asked what your least preferred and most desired birth options were? Well, this was so that you could prepare emotionally and mentally and protect yourself from the potential of experiencing an event as traumatic.

Work on the event

Working on the event itself helps you to reduce the emotional energy that is associated with the event, whether it's a past event or an imagined future event.

For a past event, this means clearing out the emotional component of the event. In doing this, you're able to recall the event, but without the emotional energy that comes with it. Sometimes the emotional component is so great that when it's cleared, your memory of the event fades and you become less clear on some of the specifics. This is important to bear in mind if you need to pursue anything after the event, for example a complaint or a legal proceeding.

As an example, let's say you had a difficult c-section experience, then working on how you feel about c-sections would go some way to letting go some of the emotional energy you're holding about this experience. Similarly, if you hate the thought of c-sections and it features as your worst birth outcome, then letting go of the emotion in advance will help you to stay emotionally strong should that be how things turn out for you. To work on this using the Head Trash Clearance Method, you would simply insert "c-section" into the mantras.

Addressing the components of the event

Here I mean the parts of the event that really affected you or *the Thing* that happened that you can't stop thinking about.

Let's continue with our c-section example. Perhaps the bit that you're struggling with is not the c-section itself, but how you were treated by the anaesthetist beforehand. Perhaps they spoke to you rudely and made you feel disrespected. So in this instance, you could use the Head Trash Clearance Method to work on "rudeness" or "disrespect" while thinking of the c-section. To be super thorough you could do both, if appropriate.

Now let's think about your upcoming birth. I'd like you to focus on those aspects of birth that have the potential to affect you. This requires you to think more about you're own emotional triggers - the things that wind you up or stress you out - and identify those which may show up during birth. If things like *respect* and *being in control* are important to you, then they have the potential to be problematic for you if you experience a situation where you're not respected or you feel you have no choice. In the context of birth, we often come across women feeling like they haven't been treated with respect or not being given any choice, and it's this treatment that is a contributing factor in how they feel about their birth. If we can loosen the power that our need for respect or control has on us, perhaps we can reduce the potential for a situation to leave a negative emotional trace in our lives.

So when you're thinking about your future birth experience, think about those aspects that you would hate to feature in your birth. Questions to ask yourself include;

- What behaviour in others would affect me? *Being disrespectful? Being rude?*
- What situations would affect me? *Breech baby? Tearing? Needing pain meds?*
- What do I want to avoid feeling? *Vulnerable? Weak?*

The answers to these questions would be things that I recommend you work on in advance of your birth. To work on them simply take the words - as I've italicised above - and insert them into the Head Trash Clearance mantras. This will help you to shed the emotional energy around those things so that if they show up on the day, you'll be better able to handle them and respond calmly.

In addition to using the Head Trash Clearance Method, I'd like to share another technique that is brilliant for trauma relief work, one that's great if you want to think about the whole event, even if you don't have many clear memories of the event.

Tapas Acupressure Technique

You might be thinking, "Hmmmm . . . the Tapas Acupressure Technique. That sounds familiar." That's because I've mentioned it before; it's the source for the TAT hand position that we use in the Head Trash Clearance Method. It's also the technique I used to help me clear the trauma of my own birth experience. Tapas Fleming, the creator of the technique, offers a number of resources at her website that are worth checking out. If you'd like to find out more about using TAT and how you can use it to help you move past trauma, visit tatlife.net.

Chapter Thirteen

Head Trash Clearance Essentials

Now I'd like to tell you a bit more about the head trash clearance method because I believe it will help you to get better results with your clearance work.

When I first started sharing it over seven years ago, I quickly learned that I needed to give people more than just the technique. I know this because of the number of emails I was receiving! You don't actually *need* any more information to be able to do effective clearance work, but it can definitely help, especially if you have an enquiring mind and are wondering things like *Why am I doing that? What does saying that mean? Why am I doing that with my hands?* Well, you get the picture! Before long, all these questions in our heads get in the way and distract us from just getting on with the job at hand. So I'd like to pre-empt this by answering some questions so that you can put your enquiring mind to rest and just crack on.

In this chapter, I'm going to share with you some of the key underlying concepts that are worth being aware of when it comes to using the Head Trash Clearance Method. It's my hope that once you understand these key concepts that not only will your questions will be answered, but you'll also be able to up your clearance game.

The Law of Opposites

The law of opposites is a cornerstone of the method and runs through it like DNA. If you want to achieve great results, it's important that you understand more about this law, and specifically how it applies to our emotional life.

The law of opposites is sometimes known as the *law of duality* and is one of the universal laws that exists, alongside laws like the *law of cause and effect*, the *law of gender*, the *law of attraction*, and the *law of vibration*. This law states that everything in the universe has its opposite: Right – Left; Front – Back; Hot – Cold; Up – Down. It not only states that everything has an opposite: it is *equal* and *opposite*. In physics, this is reflected in Newton's Third Law: For every force, there is an equal but opposite force.

I'd like you to imagine a seesaw. At one end of the seesaw is a huge boulder, the kind that Wile E. Coyote would always try and aim at the Road Runner. If you want to balance this seesaw you have to apply a force at the other end of the seesaw that equals the force being applied by the boulder. Otherwise your seesaw ain't budging! Now, let's say that you happen to come across a boulder of the exact same weight and are able to get it onto the seesaw. Your seesaw will now be in balance. Hoorah! But I'm not sure how long this seesaw will last with all this weight weighing it down. If you really want the seesaw to be in balance AND survive, you're better off removing BOTH boulders. Then it can move freely as required.

It's worth mentioning at this point that the universe is always seeking balance, so if you haven't found a boulder to balance the seesaw, the universe will kindly provide a boulder for you, thus putting this metaphorical seesaw in balance. This is why we have things like lightning and static electricity; it's the universe restoring balance. It doesn't always do this straight away, but it's always striving and moving towards it. Once enough force is applied, it springs into balance, just as we feel the atmosphere changing when a storm is building. Suddenly it all culminates in a thunderclap and lightning as the charges balance themselves out. But let's get back to our seesaw, and this time let's replace the boulders with emotions.

Let's say that you're honest person. Now, let's imagine that at one end of your seesaw you've got a boulder that represents honesty. As you're a big fan of honesty, it's a pretty big boulder. It needs to be in order to hold all the love-energy you have for it. Honesty is super important to you, and you put a lot of energy into ensuring that you're as honest as can be at all times. You love honesty so much that when other people aren't, it really annoys you. This is because you hate dishonesty. You hate it with a vengeance! It would be impossible for you to feel any other way about dishonesty. Dishonesty is not really a "meh" thing for you . . . you HATE it!

The reason you hate dishonesty as much as you love honesty is because the universe is seeking balance, and they are opposites for you. In order for you to love honesty so much, there has to be something at the opposite end that you hate at the same level. I'm assuming it's dishonesty, but it could just as easily be something like corruption, fraudulence, or immorality.

So you see, when we're looking to lighten our emotional load, the way to begin is to remove the emotional energy that exists around something. If you want to be less easily triggered by lying, dishonest cheats, then a great place to start would be clearing the hate-energy you have for dishonesty. And, for the sake of balance, you also have to clear the love-energy you have for its opposite, which might well be honesty. Otherwise, over time, the universe will seek to balance things out and will eventually re-fill your hate-energy tank. For lasting emotional relief, you need to address BOTH ends of your emotional seesaw, which will bring you to a place of neutrality (which I'll talk about in a bit).

Earlier, I said that the law of opposites runs through this clearance technique like DNA. In fact, the law of opposites manifests in two important ways:

1. Within the head trash clearance mantras
2. In our need to work on the opposite of The Thing we think we're working on

1. The law of opposites in the head trash clearance mantras

When I shared the head trash clearance mantras, you may have noticed that our ten mantras are essentially just five -the only difference being that one is a *love* mantra and one is a *hate* mantra. The reason we use two versions of this mantra is so we can clear the emotional energy from the emotional polar opposites of each one. (I'll explain more about the head trash clearance mantras in a bit, as I'm sure you're wondering why we say those things!). And, because we're doing emotional clearance work, we're using the two most powerful emotions; *love* and *hate*.

2. Our need to also work on the opposite issue

When I shared with you the 5-Step Head Trash Clearance Method, you may have noticed that Step 5 is "do the opposite." Well, this is why you need to work on the opposite issue too. As we learned above, if you don't work on the opposite of the thing you want to clear, you run the risk of being out of balance which the universe will try and fix.

If you're working on, let's say, a *fear of pain*, then you will also need to work on things like:

- Calmness around pain
- Fear of pleasure

If you're stuck trying to figure out the opposite, Google it! It can be hard to figure out what the opposite of something is, so I find doing an internet search helps me to hone in and find exactly what it is for me. The thing to bear in mind about opposites is that they're unique to each of us, and what might be the opposite of something for one person might not be for another. Think of *stress*, for example. When I've run workshops and asked for the opposite of *stress* I've received all sorts from my workshop attendees: calm, joy, happiness, clarity, content, peaceful, etc. This is personal, so just go with whatever resonates most with you. Once you've successfully worked on both ends of something, something interesting happens: you achieve *neutrality*.

Neutrality

When I first learned about neutrality, I thought it meant *feeling neutral* about something. It's easy to see why one might think that, but that's not quite it. In fact, neutrality is the opposite of polarity. And while that might not be immediately helpful, let me share some definitions of polarity to help you understand.

Polarity

1. The state of having or expressing two directly opposite tendencies or opinions, etc.
2. The presence or manifestation of two opposite or contrasting principles or tendencies.
3. The positive or negative character of a word or other item in a language.

In everyday life we come across polarity in batteries and other such electrical items, and we might hear people talk of a negative or positive charge. To be honest, this isn't a million miles away from what's going on in our bodies; our body has electrical current running through it, and the state of our health and well-being is revealed by observing whether our body is positive or negative in its electrical charge. Feel free to measure your personal electrical current with a voltmeter to see what I mean. If you're in negative, one way to switch polarity is to state affirmations and focus your mind on positive emotions and aspects of your life. This can help you to switch to a positive charge.

If we think about polarity in terms of emotions, then when we think about polar opposites, the obvious emotions that come to mind are the most powerful ones: love and hate. And so it follows that there are things we love and things we hate, and our view on those things is usually pretty fixed. If we love chocolate today, it's unlikely that tomorrow we'll hate it. So if we're to think about what the opposite of that might be, it isn't feeling nothing or neutral about something, but instead being able to choose whether we love, like, or hate it depending on the situation we're in. Let's stick with chocolate as our example since I've already mentioned it.

Let's say you LOVE chocolate! And when I say LOVE, I mean you're pretty much addicted. I mean you REALLY love it. In fact, a day doesn't go by when you don't eat any. If you see a piece of chocolate, then you'll take a bite. If you have chocolate in the house, then it won't last long because you'll end up eating it. If you're offered some, you'll say yes - you find it pretty hard to resist because you love it so much. This might actually sound familiar to you! The thing about chocolate lovers is that this is where they spend their days: in the chocolate-loving zone, wondering when they'll be able to get their next chocolate fix. It's highly unlikely that chocolate lovers would ever wander into the chocolate-hating zone.

Of course, there might well be people who HATE chocolate. I'm sure there must be! At least, let's assume there are for the purposes of my illustration. These chocolate haters will go out of their way to AVOID chocolate. They can't even bear to hear the crinkling of choco-late wrappers, let alone the smell! Now, as with our chocolate lovers, it's very unlikely that these guys will ever switch over to become chocolate lovers. They will spend their days in the chocolate-hating zone, wondering what they could possibly eat to go with their coffee.

So, what is the opposite of this scenario? What's the opposite of the idea of people being stuck at either of the polar extremes of the chocolate spectrum? It can't be feeling neutral about chocolate because, if these people did exist, they would just be sitting halfway between the lovers and the haters. So what is it?

It would be the *ability* to love chocolate (but not be totally addicted to it) AND the ability to hate it (or dismiss it). There are days when you really enjoy it, and then it might be days or weeks before you have some again. There might even be times when you're really not in the mood and you turn chocolate down! As crazy as this seems, this is someone who is experiencing neutrality in regards to chocolate. They can love it or leave it. But it's certainly not a neutral feeling. Instead, it's an ability to eat chocolate mindfully. To be able to CHOOSE when to eat it and enjoy it, rather than being stuck at the I LOVE IT, SO I GOTTA EAT IT end or the I HATE IT, DON'T EVEN WANNA SEE IT end.

When you love or hate something, you hold a lot of love- or hate-energy for it. This is the energy we see in your body's reactions. The thing is, this energy is polarising and keeps you stuck in your pre-established behaviours and thoughts. This is why you find it hard to be selfish if you think that being selfish is a bad thing, or to be disrespectful if you think respect is a good thing. Don't get me wrong, you are still capable of being selfish and disrespectful, but you won't be doing so mindfully. Instead you'll be doing so as part of a reaction that you're not really able to control. You might not even realise that you're doing it, but believe me . . . you are! We are often most guilty of the thing we hate in others.

When we clear the excess emotional energy around something, what we're actually doing is removing that energetic emotional weight in order to enable you to stand at the middle of the seesaw. From this new position, you can now easily move to either end, depending on what the situation you're in calls for. There is no resistance from your thoughts, feelings, emotions, or beliefs; you have flexibility of thought and behaviour, and the freedom to choose how to respond (freedom, choice, and flexibility!). This is neutrality: the ability to act mindfully in any given moment, with no predetermined default behaviour pattern kicking in without you thinking it or wanting it.

Here's another way to think about this: Imagine you have a bunch of emotions that you carry with you everywhere, no matter the circumstance. Let's say frustration is one of them. Imagine frustration is like a big, heavy hammer and you carry it around in your hand. Because it's in your hand, you're always using it, even if it's not required or appropriate. But you can't help it - it's in your hand. So you're frustrated that you've just missed the bus, you're frustrated that the printer is out of paper, you're frustrated that the person in front of you just ordered the last meal of the day . . . you get the picture. Everything is frustrating.

Now, how about you get yourself a tool belt? Radical, huh? Then you can put the tool down and only pick it up when you need it. You still have it with you, but it's not in your hand getting mixed up in everything you do. Having neutrality around frustration is like having it in the tool belt that enables you to lighten the emotional load that you might be carrying.

Freedom, Choice, and Flexibility

In explaining neutrality, I talked about freedom, choice, and flexibility. I'd like to dwell on this for a brief moment because understanding freedom, choice, and flexibility when it comes to our head trash can be quite enlightening. Let me share some examples that I hope explain things.

If you have a fear, let's say a fear of giving birth, then you will do everything you can to avoid experiencing birth. The lengths you go to will depend on how fearful you are. At one end, you might choose to avoid the birthing process altogether and opt for a C-section, while at the more extreme end, you might avoid becoming pregnant, or even have an abortion if you found yourself pregnant. In this example, whichever action you choose to take, while it might seem like a choice, it's not really. You are being forced into making this choice because your fear has eliminated other choices for you. If you had no fear, you would be in a position to choose from a fine platter of choices: Hospital or home birth? Induction or natural birth? Keep the baby or not? With an extreme fear of birth, you have lost the *freedom* to experience the various possibilities of birth, you are limited in *choice* in the kind of births you're open to experiencing, and you're not *flexible* in finding thinking patterns that could help you find solutions to the challenges you're facing. The same goes for any fear: we deliberately take steps to avoid doing something *because it's too scary*, so in fact we're being forced to follow a particular route of action.

The same goes for a negative emotion. Let's say you absolutely hate dishonesty in others. You wouldn't be free to be dishonest if the need came up because you hate it too much! You couldn't choose to be dishonest because, as far as you're concerned, your only option would be to be honest (not helpful if a robber in a black-and-white stripey top is asking you for the combination code for the safe) and this is all because your thinking (and hence your behaviour) isn't flexible enough to allow for times of creative dishonesty in your life.

And what about any limiting thoughts or beliefs you may have? Beliefs like *childbirth is painful*, or *the only place to give birth is in a hospital surrounded by a team of medics on standby* are likely to stop you from fully considering all the options available to you. By reducing your options at the outset, you're limiting your freedom, choice, and flexibility to respond to whatever situation ultimately presents itself. It's important to remember that just because we prepare for a particular preferred outcome, it doesn't mean we get it. Things may go off-track, and birthing is no exception. If you have the belief that *a hospital is the only place to give birth* and you end up going into labour quickly and unexpectedly at home, then your ability to respond calmly will be hugely beneficial to you. But if you're worrying about the fact that you're not in hospital, rather than allowing and accepting things to unfold at home, then you're making things emotionally harder for yourself, which will in turn impact your childbirth experience.

The same could be said of a subconscious or default pattern of behaviour. When we respond angrily to little Jonnie for accidentally spilling the milk, are we really making a decision in that moment to be angry (a choice) or is it an automatic response that we couldn't help (a reaction)? Are we able to be flexible in how we respond (i.e., not always showing anger) depending on what might be most appropriate in that moment? Often, it's our inability to act with freedom, choice, and flexibility that causes us stress and angst. By neutralising the nega- tive thought, feeling, or emotion, we restore our ability to act with freedom, choice, and flexibility, and this is what enables us to be mindful in our lives. Living mindfully not only helps us to live with less stress, but it also means we're better able to respond to what life brings us moment to moment.

Mindfully Angry

Let's see how mindful behaviour looks like when it comes to anger. I myself have witnessed a huge change in my own behaviour, which comes in very handy as a mum. Before I worked on this, I would have been one of those people who curses the house down at a huge spill, and then proceeds to be this horrible angry person for about an hour as it squirms around my system. Instead, today I'm able to respond calmly and just get on with cleaning it up and then move on to the next joyous moment that my kids will undoubtedly bring me. After all, they're just kids and they didn't do it on purpose. If they did do it on purpose, then I choose to be angry, understandably. But the key thing is that I'm choosing to show that I'm angry and that I'm in control of it.

There are times when being angry is useful and worthwhile, particularly according to my own parenting style (which is not up for debate right this moment!). Sometimes it's useful for my children to see me angry and not happy about something, but usually it's because I've *decided* to be angry. Anger is a healthy emotion that needs to be expressed, and my kids need to learn how to express their anger, so in those moments I am leading by example.

What I'm not encouraging here is no anger, ever! Bottling up emotions is only going to go one way: BADLY! Instead, what I'm suggesting is a mindful use of anger. You choose when to be angry and the level of anger you have. It's controlled and measured, as opposed to this big emotional explosion that's full of curse words and abrupt movements (slamming doors, etc.). In fact, it's quite calm, which can feel a little bit more scary, actually, even as an adult. When someone is angry and losing it (emotionally), it can be all too easy to dismiss them for "having a moment." But when the anger is delivered in a calm way, the message behind it has more impact.

The same goes with any emotion. If you can demonstrate an

emotion without losing it emotionally, people listen. Just think of those topical news programmes in which you often see heated debates (in the UK we have shows like *Newsnight* and *Question Time* for this). When someone is putting their view out there and they're losing control of their emotions, we stop listening and start noticing the emotional reaction instead. If they're able to remain calm in those moments, our attention will stay focussed on what they're saying.

The great thing about being able to do this is that you can let go of the emotion as soon as you no longer need it, rather than carrying it around for hours or days. So if I'm with my kids and the eldest has just done something silly, I show her how angry I am about what she's done and then I put the anger down and go back to being "normal" (ha! whatever that is!), which means that if I need to be present with my youngest or chatting to my partner, I'm able to do that without anger. Now, don't get me wrong - I'm not perfect at this. I still have a shed-load of emotional triggers to work on, but having spent years clearing the things that trigger my negative emotions, I'm much better able to remain present and mindful most of the time, which is a huge improvement compared to the permanent stress-fest that used to be my life experience.

The Hidden Dimensions of Head Trash

When we imagine a person in therapy, it's usually one person on a couch talking about their problem and how it's affecting them. If their problem is negative in nature, then the person on the couch is probably talking about how much they hate having this problem because of how much upset it causes them in their life.

This all sounds fair enough, doesn't it? We could say that in this particular therapy session the therapist is helping the person to explore one dimension of their problem: how it relates to themselves. In fact, they're only actually exploring half a dimension, since it sounds like they're only talking about how much they *hate* their problem. If you've been paying close attention since the start of this chapter, you've hopefully picked up on the fact that only looking at aspects we hate is missing half the picture: what about the aspects we love? Remember the law of opposites?

As we've discovered, we can't really get a great handle on a problem if we only look at one side of it. And we certainly can't fully let go of it if we only let go of half of it. If we want to clear our head trash around something we need in order to clear out the love-energy we have for it as well as the hate-energy. But it doesn't stop there.

When we open our eyes to the vastness of our emotional landscape, it's quickly evident that there is much more baggage around an emotional issue than what we've been looking at up until now: how we as individuals negatively experience the problem. We're social creatures on an overpopulated planet; whatever personal emotional challenge we have doesn't affect only us, and it would be naive to think so. It affects other people too. And the bit that psychologists have failed to explore is this: what happens to us when these other people are being affected by this thing? When you take a closer look, we get affected quite a lot, actually. We don't operate in silos; we're very much interconnected with those around us, and yet this is rarely explored in therapeutic terms.

Let's imagine that you're out with your partner, having dinner in a nice restaurant. You've just finished your starter and you're enjoying the welcome pause that comes between dishes when you notice a couple at the next table. The reason you notice them is because of the way that the husband is speaking to his wife; he seems incredibly rude and disrespectful, and is saying things to his wife that you find uncomfortable to listen to. You try to ignore it, but you're finding it quite hard to because you're wondering how on earth she's putting up with it. Your mind wanders from the lovely conversation you were having and you start imagining the things you would like to say to put him in his place.

The man at the next table continues with his disrespectful ways, this time directing them at the waiter. Upon hearing how he speaks to the waiter, you feel tension rising inside and you notice that you're starting to feel quite mad. More than anything, you want to jump to the defence of the wife or the waiter and put this man in his place. Your partner notices that you seem distracted, but you shrug it off. The thing is, you can't shrug it off. You're annoyed, and as long as you carry on hearing this man carry on like this, you get more and more annoyed and angry. This has become *your* problem.

But why? This has nothing to do with you. The man is not directing any of his rudeness or his lack of respect at you. It's the wife's and the waiter's problem. So how come this has now become your problem? Hmmm. Does this situation sound familiar? Have you ever found yourself wound up by other people's behaviour when you have no idea who they are, and when what they're doing has absolutely nothing to do with you? Well, my friend: you have just been triggered by one of the hidden dimensions of head trash!

These kinds of situations demonstrate the other dimensions to our head trash that we need to take into consideration when doing emotional clearance work; focussing solely on how a problem affects us individually isn't enough. We also need to address other aspects of the problem, aspects that we may have previously dismissed. So what are these other hidden aspects?

In all, there are five dimensions of head trash that we need to address if we are to fully let go of an emotional issue.

1. The idea or the concept of it

This is the very idea of the head trash. It's not personal and doesn't relate to anyone specifically. It's merely the concept of something.

A great example here is Depression (I deliberately use a capital D here, as I'm referring the to condition referred to as Depression, as opposed to occasional bouts of depressed feelings).

We hear Depression mentioned a lot in the context of mental health, and it frequently makes the news, often triggered by the revelations of yet another celebrity owning up to suffering from it or, sadly, choosing to end their life because of it. The ensuing discussions and debates might talk about how little support is available for sufferers or how it's so often misunderstood. When we hear Depression talked about in this way, it doesn't really have a personal angle; instead, it's being debated as a thing.

Let's say you suffer from Depression or you occasionally experiences bouts of depression or depressed feelings and you hear such a story come up on the news. How might that make you feel? It's highly probable that it would have an effect on you in some way. Maybe it would remind you of how you feel when you're depressed. Or perhaps you might feel a dark, empty feeling creep back in or be reminded of the times when you were depressed. Whatever your response, it's highly unlikely that you would hear a story of Depression on the news and not be affected in some way.

Compare that to a person who doesn't suffer from Depression who hears the same story. This person might not even notice the story when it comes on and will simply carry on doing whatever it is they're doing as the news carries on in the background. For them it's a non-event.

This is what we refer to as the first dimension of head trash: *the very idea of it*. We can't ignore the fact that simply hearing about something being discussed - depression, miscarriage, death, burglary, rape, etc. - can trigger an internal response that might include sounds or images coming to mind or physical feelings or sensations in our body. This response could be mild, or it might kick off a cascade of thoughts, feelings, and emotions that have a real impact on us.

When I was tokophobic, I was caught out by this once on the underground in London. I read a paper that had been left on the seat and it included a story of a woman who had given birth in a taxi. I cried! I had a mini-freak-out right there in the train carriage.

When we talk about this dimension of head trash, here are some examples of how we express it:

- Anger
- Depression, depressed feelings
- Childbirth, giving birth
- Pain

2. Your personal experience of it: you experiencing the head trash

This dimension of head trash is the one that we're most aware of and is the one that's usually tackled in many talking therapies: head trash and how we experience it.

Keeping with the examples I shared with you above, this dimension of head trash is expressed like this:

- Anger: me being angry, me experiencing anger

- Depression: me being / feeling depressed, me experiencing Depression / depressed feelings
- Childbirth: me experiencing childbirth, me giving birth
- Pain: me being in pain, me experiencing pain

We're all too familiar with exploring our feelings within this dimension, but perhaps the aspect we don't consider enough is how we might love this thing that bothers us. This might sound like an outlandish statement, but on some level we need to acknowledge that a small part of us loves the thing we hate. We might never want to admit this to ourselves, but we need to take a look nonetheless. Particularly if we've had this problem for years. If we didn't love it so, why haven't we gotten rid of it already?

Let's take the person who experiences bouts of depression as an example. When she's having a bad phase, she might be fortunate enough to have good friends and family who step in and help her to take care of herself. Perhaps her family will use it as an excuse to come and visit and to check up on her. On some level she will love this level of connection that her depression brings her. Deep down she might think that if it wasn't for her depressed state, she might not see her friends and family as much, so why would she stop being like this? It follows that on some level she loves it. That is not to say that any of this is conscious or deliberate, but if we are to truly let go of something, we need to recognise that there is going to be a small part of us that loves this thing too.

There are many people who choose not to overcome a phobia or an emotional challenge, even though the possibility exists for them to do so. Why would that be? Perhaps it's because of the secondary gain they receive as a result.

3. Other people being affected by the head trash

This is when other people are being affected by the head trash in question. These other people have nothing to do with you; they're just other folks who are also experiencing this emotional challenge.

Working with our examples, this is how that might be expressed:

- Anger: other people being angry / experiencing anger
- Depression: other people being depressed, experiencing depression
- Childbirth: other people giving birth
- Pain: other people being in pain / experiencing pain

By taking a closer look, we're better able to understand how other people experiencing this thing also affects you. In the restaurant scenario I shared earlier, even though these other people (the wife and the waiter) were experiencing disrespect and rudeness, you were the one who was being triggered emotionally.

It's important for us to acknowledge how the world around us affects us, even though we might not be targeted directly. If we're to live a life that's as calm and stress-free as possible, it helps if we can free ourselves from the ways other peoples' behaviour can affect and influence us, even if the behaviour isn't aimed directly at us.

Within the birthing environment, this is crucial if you are to remain in a calm mental and emotional state to avoid disrupting your hormones. You don't want to find yourself being triggered into annoyance and anger by the way a doctor or consultant speaks to a midwife in your presence, for example.

4. When you make other people experience the head trash (*to* others)

This is where things get interesting, because now we start to acknowledge the role *we* play in making other people experience head trash. This dimension is about *you making other people experience the head trash*, and how that in turn might affect you. In terms of our examples, this is how it looks:

- Anger: me making other people experience anger, me angering others, me making other people feel angry
- Depression: me depressing others, me making other people feel depressed
- Childbirth: me making other people give birth, me making other people experience giving birth

- Pain: me making other people experience pain, me inflicting pain on other people

There are different levels and aspects within this dimension that are worth exploring; after all, it's possible to make someone else experience something by accident or deliberately, just as it's possible to encourage or support them in experiencing something. Here's what I mean:

- Me *deliberately* making someone else angry: by knowingly damaging their property, by being rude to their face
- Me *accidentally* making someone else angry: by being late, by unwittingly saying something they don't agree with
- Me *encouraging* someone to stay angry: by reminding them why they're angry and reinforcing their view, by saying something I know will reignite their anger

You might have read the comment "me making other people give birth" and thought WHAT? Well in this context, it could be expressed in some of the following ways;

- Me *encouraging* or *persuading* someone else to go through with birth (a vaginal birth say instead of a c-section)
- Me *supporting* someone else in giving birth (cheerleading them and giving them high-fives and positive comments)

5. When other people or situations make you experience the head trash

Our final dimension is when other people (or situations) make you experience the head trash. In other words, this is when you're experiencing the feeling or displaying the behaviour, *because of someone or something*. This dimension acknowledges those situations in which we are actually being triggered by something:

- Anger: other people or situations making me angry, other people or situations angering me
- Depression: other people or situations making me feel depressed, other people or situations depressing me
- Childbirth: other people or situations making me give birth, other people or situations making me experience childbirth
- Pain: other people or situations making me feel/experience pain

As you can see from the second-to-last example, sometimes we need to spend a bit of time getting the phrasing right. The phrase *other people or situations making me give birth* sounds a bit weird when we first hear it, but said another way, it could be *me being induced before I'm ready*. The sense is still the same - being made to experience something. This is why I recommend that you write out your head trash clearance mantras beforehand so that you can find phrases that make sense to you.

Now, I'm quite a visual person, so to help me get my head around all of this when I was training, I created a little diagram. I've since found that the people who attend my training courses love this little picture too:

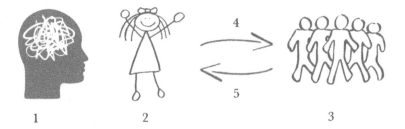

Where

1. **Head trash** - The idea of it
2. **Within** - You experiencing the head trash
3. **Others** - Other people experiencing the head trash
4. **To others** - Making other people experience the head trash
5. **From others** Other people making you experience the head trash

Even though I just shared five dimensions of head trash with you, there are in fact ten, since each one is made up of two parts: the love aspect and the hate aspect. I hope that you've now made the link between these ten aspects of head trash and the ten head trash clearance mantras.

The head trash clearance mantras

Each head trash clearance mantra relates to one of the dimensions of head trash, so by working your way through each of the dimensions, you're in fact undertaking a very thorough emotional clear-out. Then, when you also work on clearing the opposite of your head trash, you've completed the most powerful emotional clear-out possible. Not only that, but it's a deep level of work that you would not have achieved through traditional therapeutic means, simply because traditional talking therapies do not help you to let go and clear the emotional baggage that's hiding in these other dimensions. In fact, most traditional therapies just work on what's hiding in half of one dimension, as I touched on earlier. So you could say that this approach has ten times the depth of clearance. Twenty times when you acknowledge the power that's contained in clearing the opposite too. Wowsers!

I talk about all this in the "Hidden Dimensions" episode of *The Head Trash Show* podcast.

One thing to bear in mind is this: when you're doing clearance work using this technique, it's important to elicit the strongest emotional reaction possible. This will help to bring any hidden or buried emotions to the surface, which is a *good thing* for clearance work. Sometimes we don't choose the interpretation or the language that accurately reflects the actual situation, but instead choose language that will elicit the strongest emotional reaction. In this case, that might be "me deliberately making someone else angry." I would imagine that the level of resistance that pops up when you say that to yourself is pretty strong. If it is, brilliant! Use it! But perhaps the very idea that you've made someone else angry by accident leaves you feeling awful and distraught. If this is the case, it would be worth using this phrase too.

Don't be afraid to mix and match your mantras to make them work for you.

Using LOVE and HATE in the Mantras

We've already talked about how love and hate are the most powerful emotions, so when we want to do some deep clearance work, we need to apply the law of opposites to the far reaches of your head trash, which means applying it to each of the hidden dimensions.

Let me invite you to think of something emotional for a minute. No . . . that could get messy. How about you think of a wet flannel instead? Yes. Think of a wet flannel. A heavy, soggy flannel. Now imagine picking it up. How would that feel?

Heavy? Weighed down? It would affect everything it came into contact with; everything would get wet! It would be a bit of bummer wouldn't it? And not in a good way. It would be rather messy. In fact, when you think about it, this wet flannel is sort of like us when we're emotional: we feel heavy, weighed down, and a bit teary, and we affect those around us. But I digress - back to the flannel.

Let's say you wanted to make the flannel more manageable, less messy and wet, and lighter. How would you go about doing that? What would you do if you wanted to make sure that as much water came out as possible?

Did you say you'd *twist* it? In *opposite* directions? Yes! Wringing it in opposite directions would be the most effective way of removing the excess water; by wringing it to opposite extremes, we're able to remove the excess water and return it to a semi-dry state.

The same idea is at play when we use emotional opposites to remove excess emotional energy from each of the dimensions.

Let's imagine for a minute that you hate the thought of pain. Like, you really, really hate the thought of pain. In fact, you hate it so much that you'll consider having a C-section just to avoid the possibility of experiencing pain in labour. That's a lot of hate-energy right there. So if we're going to expel all that emotional energy, one of the things we're going to need to do is to LOVE pain. Like *really* love it! Love it as much as we can. Now, admittedly, if you hate the thought of pain, this is going to feel a bit weird. Loving pain? Yes! But an important thing happens when you sit and focus your thought-energy on loving pain: your resistance pops up. Or, depending on how much you hate pain, it might SCREAM up, saying things like, "No, I don't! I don't love pain; I hate it! No! No!" The more you sit with it, the more you wear your resistance down. Well, actually, you're just wringing it out. And the longer you spend with the love and hate phrases, the more you wring out the emotional energy, just like the longer your wring the wet flannel, the less wet it becomes.

Once you've gone through this process for each of the dimensions, you'll find that your hatred of pain isn't so powerful; it's lost its power and its energy. So, while you're not exactly in a place that loves it, you're no longer in a place that hates it with such vengeance. This, my friend, is that lovely place called neutrality.

I hope that this little detour of these key concepts has helped you to better understand how best to proceed. It may have also helped you to better understand yourself (which would be bonus!). In the next chapter, I'm going to answer some of the questions I'm frequently asked. This is because I like to be thorough, but also, because I'm a bit lazy, I want to reduce the emails I might get!

Chapter Fourteen

Frequently Asked Questions

I mentioned earlier that our enquiring minds can sometimes get the better of us. But also, sometime we just get stuck! So, what follows are the answers to other questions I think you might have that I may not have answered so far in the book.

You're in luck if some of the questions that you still have include;

- What can I add to my head trash clearance to do list?
- What happens when I clear head trash?
- How long does it take to notice a difference?
- Why hasn't my score gone down?

But, before I dive into that I want to quickly talk to you about your head trash clearance to-do list.

Your Head Trash Clearance To-do List

We have to-do lists for everything else in our lives, yet we neglect to have a to-do list for clearing our own mind and headspace. We have shopping lists, work project lists, household chores list, and yet the part that is the most important in ALL of this is *US*. If we're stressed, depressed, overwhelmed, or panicky, it doesn't really matter that we know where we are with our household chores, because inside we're a mess. If there's total mayhem inside our heads, surely that is the place to start, not that pile of crap that's built up near the back door. After all, we take our head everywhere with us, and it's with us until the end. Shouldn't that be the first place we start in terms of to-do lists? Of course it should.

Birth preparation is going to be one of those events in your life that is probably going to have a to-do list . . . so now is the time to add a head trash clearance section.

Adding Things to Your Head Trash Clearance To-do List

As you think about the head trash you want to clear, the first important thing to do is to notice *how you describe* your head trash in your head. For example, you might say to yourself, "I just feel really misunderstood about this and it's upsetting me." So here your head trash would be *feeling misunderstood* and/or *being upset*. If you're worried about all the work you've got to do, you might be thinking, "I've just got too much to do and not enough time to do it in." Here it would be *having too much to do* and/or *not having enough time*. If you're worried about your childbirth and you're saying, "I just can't stop worrying about the birth; what if I have complications?" then you would need to work on *worrying about birth* and/or *having complications*. At its very simplest it's as easy as that. Just use the things I've italicised above because those are the phrases you'll be inserting into the mantras.

You will need to capture these phrases somewhere that you can access easily and frequently. I put them on my phone. A notes app such as Evernote is great for this. Whenever something happens in day-to-day life that triggers me or causes an emotional reaction, I take a moment to try and figure out what it was. Then I add it to my list. I might not do the clearance work then and there, but at least it's jotted down for when I do have the time. Typically my Head Trash Clearance to-do list on my phone is two to three screens long.

Things that have been on my list include

- Fear of injections
- Being rejected, rejection
- Being in control
- Freedom, being free
- Feeling trapped, being trapped
- Responsibility, being responsible
- Being told what to do
- Being strong (and weak)

It's quite likely that you will have a pretty long list of things you need to work on. This is completely normal, especially if you haven't spent any time doing emotional clearance work before. Whatever you do, don't let your list overwhelm you. If it does, add *overwhelm* to the top of it and work on that first.

If you don't have a reasonably long list and you haven't done anything like this before, then there might be a few things going on:

Your head is in a bit of a tangle and you can't quite see the wood for the trees

If this is you, it's probable that it all feels a bit overwhelming, and trying to identify any one thing is just too hard. In these situations I urge you to sit with your feelings for a while and be aware of the thoughts that come up. Another approach is to think in super broad terms just to help take some of the emotional energy out of what you're feeling. So things like *work stresses, birthing fears, body-related anxieties,* etc. This can help you break things down so that the things hiding within start to show their face.

This is one of the reasons I've provided you with the Childbirth Fears audio session to accompany this book; it will help you to break down your head trash into pieces so that you can better understand what's going on.

You're in denial

Yup! You're doing a fantastic self-sabotaging job persuading yourself that you don't actually have anything to work on. I've seen this before; in fact, I've got the T-shirt myself somewhere! And on some level you're right. If you're content, calm, and not really affected negatively by all the happenings of life around you, then you probably don't need to do this. But if you're stressed, struggle with confidence or self-esteem, procrastinate, avoid people, places, or actions because of something, have trouble sleeping, eat or drink too much, have health issues, live day-to-day with things like guilt, anger, or resentment . . . well, you get the picture! All this stuff is a sign that you have things that need attention. So if this is you, then you might need to have a word with yourself because you're probably in denial on some level.

You're sorted!

You're an enlightened being who emanates peace and love. You're never stressed and never have a bad word to say about anything. In fact, people are drawn to you for your calming presence and your wise words. Yay for you!

What Should I be Adding to My Clearance To-do List?

I don't know about you, but I like things to be organised and to have structure, so I'm naturally drawn to categorising things and putting similar things together. This might be head trash, but I prefer to think of it as one of the quirks of my personality. Who knows? When I was going through my own learning journey around head trash clearance, I wanted to know what kinds of things I could add to my list: what *categories* of things? I was confused at the beginning (I had a lot of crap taking up space in there!), and I needed some pointers to help me figure it out. Now, I'm not saying that's you, but it might be. So if you like categories and things to be in neat piles, this part of the book is for you!

Broadly speaking, there are three types of things that you can add to your head trash clearance to-do list:

1. Emotional triggers
2. Emotions
3. Values

There is so much I could write on all of this, but I'm going to keep it brief because this book is about birthing preparation. So I'll share the aspects of these things and how that relates to birthing preparation.

Emotional triggers

Your emotional triggers are those things that trigger the emotional reactions within you. Here are some examples:

- People *lying* to you triggers your *anger*
- *Seeing pregnant women* triggers your *fear of pregnancy*
- *Being told what to do* triggers your *feeling out of control*
- *Seeing a needle* triggers your *fear of injections*

Working with your emotional triggers is a really powerful way of minimising the occurrence of some of the negative emotions in your life. By addressing the things that make you feel fearful, you are able to reduce the fear you experience. The same goes for the things that make you feel stressed or anxious.

Great questions to ask yourself are:

What situations make me [insert emotion]?
What behaviours in others makes me [insert emotion]?

Answering these questions can uncover many of your emotional triggers for a wide variety of things, and if you take the time to work on each of these triggers then you'll notice a huge shift in your emotional well-being.

Emotions

These are the emotions that arise as a result of getting triggered. When we work on an emotion directly, it doesn't mean that you won't experience it ever again; it simply means that if you currently have a backlog of trapped emotion, then you can release it, which should provide some short-term relief.

A great way to think about this is to think of an overflowing sink. The tap is on and there's water going everywhere. It's all a bit overwhelming. The water coming out of the tap represents the emotion that's being triggered by the tap being on (being lied to, seeing a needle, etc.). As long as the plug is still in, the sink (your system, your body) is holding on to that emotion. In this situation, to stop the overflowing mess, we can either turn the tap off (work on the emotional trigger) or take the plug out (clear the backlog of trapped emotion). Sometimes it's just quicker and easier to pull the plug; if anything, it gives you a bit more breathing space to deal with turning the tap off.

Working directly with emotions is very useful during labour and birth. You might be overcome with fear at something and you just want the fear to be out of your body so that you can restore balance to your hormones and so that your body can get back to birthing your baby without distraction.

*** Too Much Information Alert ***

During my first childbirth, I was at the point in labour where my daughter's head was crowning. I had been through two contractions but she still hadn't come out. My midwife had said that if she didn't come out on the next contraction, the ambulance guys in the lounge would have to take me into hospital. There was no way I wanted that to happen. In that moment I realised that I had a fear: I was fearful of the ring of fire. I'd heard it was really painful. I realised that this was blocking me from fully pushing her out and letting my body go. So in the time I had before the next contraction (two minutes or so) I cleared my fear of the ring of fire. She came out in the next contraction. Goodness knows how my birth would have gone if I wasn't able to clear my fear in that moment. I dread to think!

A good time to clear emotions is when you're in the thick of it, experiencing them. If you're overcome with emotion and would like to return to a calmer state, going through the clearance process is a great way of doing that. I used this when I was being monitored at the hospital when I had flown past my due date. The whole situation was a tad stressful and I knew if I was lying there stressed, this would affect my baby and hence the readings on the machines. So I spent my time clearing stress from my body. This helped me to stay calm in the moment, which was invaluable.

Your values

Your values are what you value as important in life. Our values tend to be responsible for most of our emotional stress, and because they're so important to us, we're much more open to being offended or affected by other people's behaviour. This is especially true with people who don't share our values and who dare to tread all over them. When someone behaves in a way that conflicts with our values, it can really hit us hard and we often take their behaviour personally. If we can work on clearing the emotional energy contained in our values, it can go a long way to helping us to be less emotionally unsettled in day-to-day life.

There's a lot more I could say about how our values contribute to head trash, but I think that's a separate book! I prefer to stay focussed on the job at hand, which is preparing you for childbirth.

For example, if one of your values is respect and you feel that you're not being treated with respect by your healthcare professionals during your labour, this will trigger quite a strong emotional reaction in you. You will suddenly have a lot of excess emotional energy that needs to come out, which will not be a good thing for the smooth progression of your labour. This sudden arrival of emotional energy will disturb your hormones and wreak havoc on your ability to stay in the birthing zone. Much better to pre-empt this by clearing your values in advance. That way, even if people tread all over your values, you won't have such a strong emotional reaction.

Working on your values won't *change* your values; it simply takes the emotional intensity out of them. This enables you to defend your position much more calmly and clearly without being overwhelmed by emotion.

What Happens When I Clear Head Trash?

As I've already mentioned, your body is heavily involved in your emotional life. We experience emotions through our body; that's how we know we're being emotional - we're *feeling* stuff! I've also talked about how easily emotions can become trapped. Well, guess where they get trapped? In our body! This means that when we're having an emotional clear-out, we might notice stuff happening in our body as the emotional energy is being released.

You might notice things like . . .

- Tingling sensations in your body as you release the energy from where it's being stored.
- A shift in bodily sensations as you go through the clearance mantras. For example, you might start noticing a tingling around your tummy. This then shifts to create a feeling of heartburn, which then becomes a burp you feel rising, finishing with an actual burp.
- Big sighs or yawns as you clear the emotional energy. I call these "hippo yawns" because for me they're much bigger than my normal yawns.
- Cleansing tears coming out of your eyes as the emotional

stress released. This is not the same as crying; these are more likely to be cleansing tears. That is not to say you won't cry or sob, though, as that's possible too. This is pure emotion that you're releasing, so don't be scared by it.

Whether you experience any of this or not it doesn't matter. Either is fine. We're all different.

But I know the question you're dying to ask me is actually the next one...

How Long Does it Take to Notice a Difference?

In terms of the thing that you're working on, the change can happen instantly. Whether you *notice* the change instantly is something else. Depending on what you're working on, it might be that you need to be in a trigger situation before you know whether you've experienced a shift. For some people it might take days for them to notice. Also, because the change happens deep within, you soon forget that this thing actually bothered you, so you forget to check in with yourself. Let me share a story that I hope will illustrate this.

I've mentioned already that I used to have a fear of needles and injections. Well, this fear was off the scale. Ever since I can remember the sight of needles would freak me out. As a child I remember regularly fainting at the doctor's when I had to have a blood test.

As an adult, I would be overcome with panic and anxiety in the lead-up to an injection, even over the days leading up to it! I once needed to have a medical examination as part of my work, which included an injection first thing one morning. I became incredibly faint and never really recovered that day. When I eventually got back to work later that morning I couldn't even walk across the car park, and by lunchtime someone had to drive me home. Ridiculous!

When I trained in Neuro-Linguistic Programming (NLP) with Paul

McKenna, one of our days' training was on phobias. We could choose to work on any sort - needles, small spaces, spiders, snakes, public speaking. At the beginning of the day, Paul spent some time showing us what we'd be doing using needles as his demonstration. We were in a room of about a hundred and fifty people and I was six rows back. As I sat there watching him hold the needle on stage, I could already feel my panic rising; my palms were getting really sweaty and I could feel that I was losing control of my emotions. I thought I might cry. He wanted a person to do his demo on. Half of me wanted so badly to be rid of this, but I couldn't bring myself to raise my hand; I didn't want to get any nearer to the needle in his hand. I nearly ran out crying. Crazy, right? I mean REALLY crazy! What kind of a response is that?

I went to the needle phobia group and we spent an hour or so working on our phobia. I did really well; by the end of the hour, I was able to hold a needle against my arm and not lose the plot. This was progress! But alas, it was short-lived. The time soon came to have another injection. I remember thinking, "Hey this is cool. I'm not scared." But despite this my arm was really tense. So tense that the injection was really painful. It was like in my head I was saying, "This is fine, there's nothing to be scared of. It won't hurt." Then BAM! It hurt! And my fear came right back.

Fast-forward a few years, and I had not long learned the technique the Head Trash Clearance Method is based on. I'm at a hospital for one of my early prenatal appointments. Quite early on in the appointment I'm told that I need to have some injections. Immediately my eyes pop out on sticks and my jaw drops to the floor. I explain that no one told me that I would be having injections and that I normally need time to prepare. This was a bit of a lie. All I would have done was spent the last twenty-four hours in total and utter panic. The nurse looked at me and said, "Oh, don't worry, it's not straightaway, we have to get all the needles ready first."

Gulp!

"ALL THE NEEDLES READY?!"

And with that she opened the door, showed me a seat in the corridor, and asked me to wait.

At this point, I was pretty much on the verge of a full freak-out party and was heading for delirium. But then I remembered. I had just trained in this new therapy, and on the training course it had been made pretty clear that this technique ate fears for breakfast. I remember thinking - no let me re-phrase that - I remember talking to Reflective Repatterning as if it were floating up above in the corridor and pointing to it saying "Ha! Let's see what you can do with this, then!".

I didn't have long, so I did the super-short version. I had barely finished when the nurse called me back in. She must have remembered my reaction from before because she asked if I was scared of needles. Before I could formulate my answer, I calmly responded, "No. Not anymore." In my head I did a double-take: *NO?! Not anymore? Who said that? This was freaking me out. Did I just say "no"?*

"Oh, that's good," she replied.

What happened next was weird. Weird in that it was different from how my injection appointments usually went. I was shown my seat next to the table with all the needles on it. Was I bothered? No! I calmly offered my super-relaxed arm. Then I noticed that I was really struggling. Struggling with the fact that I was calm and OK. In fact, the most noticeable thing I was feeling was apprehension. There was no fear, though. I just wasn't sure how this was going to go. I ended up talking through the injections (I'm quite chatty when I'm relaxed!), and in no time at all it was all over. Just like that. It was such a non-event. I didn't faint. I didn't hyperventilate. I didn't even break into a sweat. Nothing. I just sat there calmly being OK.

But the story doesn't end there. Due to having a certain blood condition, I had to have injections at most of my midwife appointments, which was probably monthly. For some reason I had a different midwife at each appointment, but the funny thing is, every single one said the same thing to me after each of my injection appointments: "I don't think I've ever given an injection to such a calm person before." Seriously? Ha! If only they knew. The injection gods were messing with my head, that's for sure!

Let's fast-forward a few years to my last pregnancy. When I sailed right past my due date and was hurtling towards my induction date, I decided to go for an acupuncture appointment. I never really stopped to think it through until I was lying on the couch and the acupuncturist asked if I had a fear of needles. I'd not really considered it and I had to stop and think about it for a while. I remembered that yes, I used to have a fear of ONE needle going into my body, but LOTS of needles; where did I stand on that? *How come I was lying here offering my body up as pincushion? What was I doing? Was I scared?* I gave this some thought, almost like I was searching my mind to check for any traces of fear lurking in the corners. Eventually I came to the conclusion that I wasn't scared and that this was totally fine. And that is my story of how I overcame my fear of needles.

If only I could take you back to the day that I did the clearance work. On that day I spent about five minutes doing the clearance work and I only had time to do *two* of the head trash clearance mantras: *I love needles and injections* and *I hate needles and injections*. The clearance work happened instantly. I knew this because I was walking straight into a trigger situation. Unlike my NLP experience, this time the clearance happened in my mind *and* my body. My subconscious mind was ahead of me that day when it responded more quickly than my conscious mind was able to, which was left confused by what had happened. My body had also experienced the shift immediately; my arm was completely relaxed, which meant that I didn't even notice the needles going in.

Now, I'm not saying you can expect that kind of speed with all things that you work on. A fear of needles is quite specific, and for me it wasn't tied to anything else, like a fear of blood, for example. Most things we work on will tend to be more complex than that, and they will need unpicking and untangling so that you can get to the root of it.

A *fear of childbirth* can hold and hide so much. There might be strands of medical fears (including a fear of needles), fears around losing control or losing dignity (which might include things like a fear of being ignored by a doctor), fears around responsibility or motherhood, fear of pain; my goodness, the list goes on! So in a situation like this, you would need to work on all of these component elements for you to notice a change in terms of the bigger thing. And, depending on how much emotional energy there is to clear you might need to revisit your clearance. Our emotional system can only take so much clearance in one go. It needs time to process what you're doing. So be prepared to revisit things if you need to.

What I want to make clear in sharing this story is the speed of the change in terms of how quickly it *can* occur. What is less speedy is the time it takes to untangle your fears so that you can actually name them, and then the time it takes to clear them. Most things take between five and twenty minutes to clear, but then you have to work on the opposite. Just like going to the gym, it's not an overnight thing, especially if you have a number of fears and you're not quite sure what they are.

When I'm working with my clients, they often feel so confident using the technique that they get on with the clearance work themselves; most of them choose to spend their time with me unpicking their head trash and trying to figure out what is hiding in there. This is why I've shared with you lots of typical fears that I come across. I hope that in reading them in black and white you are able to figure out which ones are yours.

I had my injection experience in my first trimester, and it was on the back of this experience that I realised I could apply this technique to my other childbirth fears. It inspired hope in me that I could actually let go of my fears and that it would work. It did, but it took me a while. I must have spent the entirety of my second trimester doing fear-clearance work, but by the time I reached my third trimester, my fears had dropped so much that I decided to change my birth plan from a hospital birth with a C-section back-up to a natural home birth.

By the way, I've made a Fearless Birthing Meditation if you'd like to release your fear of needles and injections. You can find that here www.fearfreechildbirth.com/product/fear-injections-needles/

Why Hasn't My Score Gone Down?

If after doing a clearance session your SUD score hasn't gone down, there are three possibilities:

1. You're measuring the wrong thing
2. You need a deeper level of clearance
3. You've revealed a new layer to your head trash

You're measuring the wrong thing

This is something that a lot of people do. Let me share an example of a client I was working with. We decided to work on clearing her feelings of overwhelm that accompanied her tokophobia. At the beginning she rated her overwhelm at fifteen out of ten. When I asked her at the end what her rating out of ten was she said it was still high, more than ten. When I asked her to tell me more, she explained she still had a high level of fear about birth. She was now measuring her fear of birth, whereas we were working on her feelings of overwhelm. When she focused on her overwhelm, she decided that it had dropped to a seven. This is an easy mistake to make, so make sure you're being consistent with what you're measuring.

You need a deeper level of clearance

Basically, this means that you need to go back and do some more, or to put it another way: stay longer with some of the mantras while holding the TAT position. You'll know if this is you because you will still have quite intense feelings about the *exact same issue*. So if you've just been working on *being lied to*, and you still feel a nine or ten after being lied to, then you need to go through the clearance again. Check that your mantras have had the head trash added correctly and that they make sense to you. Then go through them again. Sometimes we just need to revisit them because our system is only ready to offload a certain amount of crap at a time. It may be that you need to add some new mantras that are unique to the thing you're working on.

I did this when I was clearing my cat allergy. I wanted to let go of the emotion I had around my cat allergy so I worked on "feeling itchy, scratchy and wheezy". I HATED feeling itchy, scratchy and wheezy from being with cats! When it came to the mantra "making other people itchy, scratchy and wheezy", it just didn't make sense to me. So instead I directed it towards the cats. My new mantra became "I love making cats itchy, scratchy and wheezy" and of course the equivalent hate mantra. The release that I felt while clearing those two mantras was incredible. I think I went from sobbing to laughing uncontrollably and doing that clearance pretty much cleared my cat allergy. I still have the occasional cat that gets me going, but the intensity of my symptoms has dropped significantly.

You've revealed a new layer to your head trash

This is a slight variation on the first, but it does have a subtle difference. Let's say you began by working on how you felt as a result of someone treating you in a certain way. Perhaps you were frustrated at how someone was ignoring you. When you connected to that *moment of being ignored* and tuned in to how you felt, you decided that you felt *frustration*. And out of a score of one to ten, you were nine/ten frustrated.

Let's say that after doing the clearance work, you connect back to that *moment of being ignored*. You tune in to it and how you're feeling, and you decide that you're still at a nine/ten. At this point it's important to be clear on WHAT you're measuring, because it's possible that's changed and you've revealed a new layer of head trash. So a good question at this point might be, "how frustrated do I now feel about being ignored?". And it may well be that your response to this question is, "It just makes me so angry!" Well, now you're feeling angry and not frustrated. And guess what you need to do next? Work on clearing the anger!

In this scenario, we've revealed the next layer, which is anger. There may well be other layers that reveal themselves too, and in fact this is quite normal. It's rare for your head trash to be this one isolated thing. Usually we have these interconnected layers that need to be peeled back one by one. Our emotions are complex and intertwined. When clearing one, you're creating space for another one to rise to take its place. Be OK with this and just continue with your clearance work. The more you clear, the easier it gets.

Chapter Fifteen

Preparing For Birth

Why Prepare for Birth?
Birth is an incredibly powerful life event that deserves preparation.

Imagine you've booked a once-in-a-lifetime holiday. And then just suppose that once you booked it, you completely forgot about it until the week before. During the week before you'd probably be in a blind panic, frantically figuring out what you want to do and where you want to visit while you're there. *Do I want a hire car or not? Should I plan to do a day trip over to that beautiful waterfall?* Or, worse still, you get back and realise that there was all this stuff you didn't know about that you would've liked to have done or visited, only now it's too late. You're never going to be able to go through that experience again. What would that be like?

Many women approach birth in this way. Perhaps they work until a couple of weeks before their due date and then spend their limited time off buying baby clothes and prams or decorating the nursery. Or maybe they decide to buy a birthing book at thirty-five weeks to start getting their head around things. Well, I'm sorry to say that this is all a bit late in the day. Especially if you want have the most positive experience possible. Rocking up late to the party and winging it just isn't going to cut it when it comes to childbirth, not to mention that you'd miss out on all the excitement in the lead-up. Apparently people get more pleasure from *looking forward* to their holiday than the actual time they spend on it. That's how great planning and preparing can be; *better than a holiday*!

Birth preparation is something that doesn't get enough focus. I don't mean to lay blame anywhere by saying this: it's a simple case of we don't know what we don't know. Let's think back to the holiday scenario. You're not going to know about that wonderful weekend market on the river, or the beautiful waterfall that looks like the face of Jesus, or the statue that's been swallowed by a tree if you don't spend time researching your destination in advance. Once you've savvied up, you can then decide for yourself what you want to do. This is much easier to live with than a life of regret narrated by phrases that start with "I just wish I'd . . . "

Getting savvy is a huge part of birth prep, but mindset is just as important and both of these take time. It will take time for you to understand the various birth choices you're facing. It's going to take time for you to practise using various mindset tools and to find the ones that you get on well with. I urge you to give yourself this time and start preparing as early as you can. The kind of preparations you choose to undertake will have a lot to do with the kind of person you are. If you're a very practical person, you'll probably take the practical approach. If you're very active and love your exercise, then you'll probably focus your energy on physical activities that will keep you fit during pregnancy and help to prepare you for birth. If you're spiritually inclined, you'll probably be drawn to spiritual preparations.

One often-missed aspect, though, is the emotional preparation. Perhaps this is because it's not immediately obvious that it's required, or because we're not sure how to prepare emotionally. If things don't go well, your childbirth and labour has the potential to be the source of tremendous emotional pain for years to come. You owe it to yourself and your baby to do your homework and work towards having a positive experience as best you can, despite your efforts not guaranteeing the outcome. There are many women who spend lots of time preparing for their ideal birth and it doesn't go the way they'd hoped. But the time spent planning is not wasted. When things start to divert from their desired course, these women are much better placed to cope with how things are changing, and tend to be able to make decisions required during the birth that they're happy with later. This goes a long way in helping women to feel more in control of their childbirth.

I'd like to focus on those aspects of birth preparation that have a bearing on your emotional well-being in the lead-up to, during, and after your birth. My objective is to help you to have a positive birthing experience that will fill you with joy every time you think about it until your last breath. This means I'm less interested in you having the nursery bedding sorted or deciding which pram you should buy.

There is a very important point to make here about preparing for birth. I like to compare it to playing poker. An experienced poker player who knows all the tricks isn't guaranteed to win. We all know this. Who knows what cards will be drawn? It's luck of the draw. But - and this is a great BIG BUT - the poker player is far more likely to win, than the person who has no clue about playing poker.

Preparing for birth is a bit like poker in that respect. You can prepare until the cows come home, but all you're really doing is stacking the odds in your favour. There are no guarantees in birth. It's not just you doing it; it's your baby too, and they might be a trouble-maker or a rebel. If they want to leave their head at funny angle and get stuck, or stick their elbow out at the last minute, there's not a whole lot you can do about it. You've just got to suck it up buttercup! This is why the mental and emotional prep is so important. It helps you to cope with these curveballs.

Prenatal Classes

Prenatal classes can be an invaluable source of information and support during your pregnancy and in the lead-up to your childbirth. There are different types of classes you can take, from the very narrowly focussed ones provided by hospitals that simply educate you on the various birth options available to you within a hospital environment, to broader classes such as those put on by the National Childbirth Trust (NCT) here in the UK. There are also hypnobirthing classes and home birth classes, so be sure to seek out ones that are available in your area. Prenatal classes can also be a great source of friends and support during your pregnancy and following the birth, so consider whether you want a one-off class or a series of classes that offer you the opportunity to build relationships with other attendees.

Many parents choose to do prenatal classes in the last trimester. I did. During my first pregnancy it took me that long to feel ready for them, but I think that was because I was so focussed on my fear-clearance work that I never could have contemplated it sooner. But it seems to be a common pattern. When I asked the NCT, a UK-based charity that puts on prenatal classes for parents, why they suggest doing classes in the last trimester they said that many women say it feels "more real" in the third trimester, which is why they prefer to finish a course later in their pregnancy. Earlier on, their preference is to simply have information.

But I do think there's a case for starting earlier. Sophie Messager, who was inspired to become a doula after her birthing experience, says:

> *Starting antenatal classes earlier allowed me to really think and mature my decision about what I wanted (and not wanted) for the birth. It opened my mind to think about aspects of birth I didn't even know existed. It made me want to find out more, and to read more and to talk to more people, and completely changed the course of my experience for the better. I now know almost for certain that I would have had a completely different (and less positive) experience had I waited until the later part of my pregnancy.*

We are all starting our pregnancy journey from different places so it's important you do what's right for you. But procrastination and avoidance is not necessarily "doing what's right." Emotionally speaking, the sooner you start to embrace this transformational phase in your life the better.

Preparing the Mind

There are two aspects to this. Or at least there are in my world. There's the *mental* preparation and the *emotional* preparation. Preparing emotionally and mentally for childbirth can take time, but because we're all starting from different places, it's difficult to say how long. As with a marathon, mental and emotional preparation is an important part of the training, and different people will need different training regimes depending on their mental and physical state. Once you start the work, you may well come to realise that you really should've started sooner. Conversely, you can't start too early with this stuff; coming to grips with your mental and emotional well-being is something we could all do with, pregnant or not.

For me, the difference between *mental* and *emotional* is the subtle difference between *using the mind* and *what happens in the mind*. For example, if we think of a water wheel, the emotions are what passes through the water wheel, but the wheel itself is the mind.

Mental preparations are about learning to use and control the mind so that if negative emotions show up, we know how to deal with them. It's about knowing what to do to help us get back into a good emotional place.

Emotional preparations are about going upstream, taking a look at the emotions that make up our stream, and then taking a closer look to better understand the negative ones that keep showing up. If we're always happy, content, and confident, there probably isn't much need for us to take a look. But if we're constantly battling feelings of anxiety, fear, stress, guilt, shame, or any other murky emotions, then it would be fair to say that something is going on in our lives that needs a closer look. That's not to say that if you experience negative emotions something is wrong, but if you find that you experience these emotions a lot for no obvious or apparent reason, then that warrants attention.

Preparing emotionally means doing what you can to get your emotions to a good place so they can support you and not hinder you. This is what most of this book is about so I won't go crazy here, but it's about ensuring that you feel confident and positive towards your birth and not fearful and anxious. If you can address the causes and triggers of your negative emotions then you're less likely to experience them during birth. You don't have to limit this work to the negative emotions that are linked to birth; you can go much broader. The earlier you start this kind of work the better, because it will help you to maximise the moments you're able to marinate your baby in positive emotions, which can only be a good thing.

This can feel like a mountain to climb, so another way to help you in the birthing moment is to do the mental preparation, which will give you the tools and techniques to better manage the emotions (and decisions) that do pop up. You might not have the time, inclination, or expertise to do the emotional work required, but you probably have what it takes to learn some key mindset techniques to help you on the Big Day.

There are plenty of ways to manage your mindset, so it's important to spend time practising a few to find the ones that work for you. Common mindset techniques include:

Breathing: by focussing on our breath we're able to bring our mind to the present, limit the negative mind chatter, and prevent negative emotions taking hold. There are many breathing techniques that can help you and it's important to have a go at using them so that you can find one that works for you. Breathing is also a powerful way to relax the body and the mind so it can be used to bring you back to a good place should you wander.

Self-hypnosis: by taking ourselves into a hypnotic trance, we're able to minimise the interference from the outside and stay in the birthing zone, thus limiting the impact of mind chatter and negative emotions. Many hypnobirthing tracks can help you to stay in a relaxed state during birth, but again, it may take you time to find one that works for you. There may be certain aspects to tracks that annoy you - the music or the accent - so spend time finding ones you like and that you know work well for you.

Chanting: this is a great way to focus the mind on something, again to limit internal negative chatter. Some people use this very successfully. You can buy chanting albums which can also act as background music for your birth. Deva Premal have lots of albums that would work well here. You may have heard their music at yoga classes.

Head trash clearance: if difficult emotions pop up on the Big Day, just bat them away! This will only work for you if you've already done some of the emotional preparation work and if you're familiar enough with the technique to be able to use it without thinking too much. This is the value of practise.

During my first birth at the point of transition, I remember clearing a lot of fears. I don't remember what they were, but I do remember having to let the midwives know that if they heard me talking to myself and putting my hands up around my head, that they were to leave me alone; I was in fear clearance mode!

At one point, my midwife told me that "it" was close. OMG! This was it! Suddenly it all felt very intense and my baby's head was crowning. I had two contractions but the head didn't come through. My midwife told me that if my baby's head didn't come out in the next contraction that I would need to be taken into hospital (I had ambulance guys in the lounge on standby). In my mind, there was NO WAY that I was going into hospital. NO WAY whatsoever.

I went inward. I needed to do this. *What was stopping me? Why wasn't my baby's head coming through?* And then it came to me. Fear. I was scared of the pain of the ring of fire. If you haven't heard of the *ring of fire*, then let me enlighten you. It's the burning sensation that can sometimes accompany the stretching of the perineum as the baby comes out of your body. Lovely! Well, the thought of that was freaking me out and on some level I knew I was holding back because of that fear. So in the limited time I had before the next contraction (two minutes tops I reckon!) I cleared my fear of the ring of fire. In the next contraction she came out. My baby was here! I daren't imagine how that might have turned out if I went into hospital.

With many of these, the trick is to minimise the potential for the mind to come to life during labour and birth. The body needs to be in the driving seat, so you're either looking for techniques to keep the mind at bay so the body can stay in control, or for ways to quickly calm the mind and your emotions so that the body can get back into the driving seat. Different things will work for different people, so take the time to find one that will work for you.

Things Going Off Plan

One fear that crops up with women time and time again is that they will experience complications. *Complications.* So much can be contained in that one word. So what is meant by it? Complications don't necessarily mean things going tits up and scary. It can simply mean things not going according to plan.

It reminds me of the definition of weeds: *weeds are just plants that are in the wrong place.* They're not a certain type of plant, just NOT the one you want in that particular place. The same could be said of birth. Take, for example, the person who wants a home birth, but gets a hospital birth because of the additional monitoring that's required for her particular situation. Yet a hospital birth with lots of monitoring could be someone else's desired birth. Or just as some women choose to have a C-section and others end up needing one. Of course, certain types of complications do take us into the scary category, and it's these that make this fear so real for women. To help us deal with this fear in a practical and useful way, it's worth doing some prep work in advance.

A great place to start is to call it something else. Something that feels less scary and that's not loaded with negativity. This makes it easier to think about without getting emotional because, as we know, emotion has a tendency to cloud our judgement. I prefer to talk about things going "off plan" instead. This includes complications of the scary variety, but also includes some of the more mundane aspects of birth that might affect how we feel during labour, which can't really be called "complications" yet still hold the power to distract us from our birthing zone.

For example, if your mum said she was going to be there, but at the last minute is/becomes ill and can't make it. Or you really wanted your home water birth, but that day the cat decides to paw the side of the birthing pool and deflates it. Or you really wanted your hospital birth, but things happened so quickly that you end up birthing at home. These things would hardly be called complications, yet they have the potential to really throw you off guard emotionally. If we just prepare ourselves for complications we'd miss half the picture and not consider everything that has the potential to disrupt our birthing zone mindset.

If you can prepare emotionally for things going off plan, then you'll be much better placed to respond flexibly and calmly on the Big Day. This mindful focus on boosting your emotional resilience will limit the potential of things veering into the scary category. At the very least, you're increasing your chances of maintaining a healthy emotional response, which will go a long way to help you think positively about your childbirth experience. Many women report having unplanned C-sections that were incredibly positive experiences. They credit the way they prepared and being able to maintain emotional composure throughout as being what helped them claim their positive childbirth experience.

Grace's Story

Let me share with you Grace's story. Grace worked on her fears during her pregnancy and she credits doing that work with helping her have a positive birth experience, despite all her worst fears coming true.

"I am a Pediatric ER nurse and have seen some horrific genetic

abnormalities and other things that no mother would ever wish on her child. That being said, I started out my pregnancy in a blissful ignorance that anything could possibly go wrong with MY pregnancy/birth. Thankfully, I was hungry for as much information as I could soak in on natural childbirth. When I came across your podcast the idea of dealing with fears before they arose was rather new to me. Initially I had a hard time digging up the fears that I had. I also felt rather silly going through the five steps of clearing my fears, so I didn't bother at first. It wasn't until I was about six months along that the fear of a C-section persisted in my dreams.

About a year and a half before I found out I was pregnant, my sister had her first baby. Her story was quite horrific. Her baby was breech and she ended up needing an emergency C-section. She was devastated. I didn't realize how worried I was about this very thing happening to me until that point. More than anything, I wanted an all natural labor and birth outside of a hospital. I had a birthing center picked out and was ecstatic to experience labor and birth in its most raw form. After several weeks of digging out and identifying my fears, the fear of having to go to a hospital and worst of all having a C-section kept showing up. I will say that I had to work on this fear daily and although it became easier and easier to manage my head trash, this one was the most difficult.

When I started using your Head Trash Clearance Method consistently (every other day or so) I started feeling less stressed about the idea. I think it was step three that got me really analyzing my fear. More specifically saying "C-sections are a wonderful thing" and "I love C-sections." When I would repeat these things, I would realize that they were true! C-sections ARE a wonderful thing and if I were in need of one I would love C-sections. Looking back I am so thankful for this amazing medical intervention because there is a good chance that my baby would have died without it! Hindsight is 20/20 right?! I think in the end, I recognized my fear as irrational and turned it into something to be thankful for.

My labor contractions began at 6am. They were small period like cramps and I didn't think much of them at first. I went about my day, even went to the gym and attempted to workout until I stood up and felt a little gush of something (it was my water leaking out). After that my contractions became a little stronger but stayed about five minutes apart. I was elated! I was going to meet my baby so soon! I felt nothing but joy and although at times I was uncomfortable, I didn't have any trouble running a few errands, packing some items for the birthing center, eating some lunch and then relaxing and waiting for my husband to get home. He arrived home around 4pm and we headed to the birthing center about an hour away. By this time my contractions were about three to four minutes apart and pretty strong.

Again, my fears and worries that I had experienced during my pregnancy were nowhere to be seen! We arrived to the birthing center around 5:30pm and we were shown to an exam room. They confirmed that the fluid I was leaking slowly was indeed amniotic fluid. My midwife felt my stomach and decided that baby was head down. She then asked me if she could check my dilation. I said yes and she stated I was four cm dilated. I was a bit disappointed that I wasn't further along, but still too excited to care much. After checking me, she said she felt something odd, possibly a hand over the baby's head and most likely nothing to worry about, but suggested that we get an ultrasound to confirm. 30 minutes later we were at the hospital down the road. My fears of having to go to a hospital were rearing their ugly heads and using meditation and your clearance method, I was able to keep them in check. The ultrasound technician came in and my husband and I were all smiles, still excited about this day we've been waiting for for so long.

The next words I heard came to me like a huge punch in the stomach, "breech." My worst fears were unfolding right before my eyes and I felt more than helpless to control them. Over the next few hours my husband and I would experience and endure the very things we didn't want in our birth, IVs, monitors, Epidurals, NPO status (no food or drink), hospital personnel in our room constantly and so much more.

For the first hour or so I have to admit that I was frantic and I felt so very helpless to defend myself against my fears. There was part of me that wanted to insist on delivering my breech baby vaginally. When I brought this up to my midwife she was quick to remind me that it could be very dangerous seeing as the providers who were caring for me were not trained in delivering breech. I felt that I had no choice but to go ahead with the few options I had left. It all happened so incredibly fast that it did take me a while to realize that I was losing control of my mind and allowing myself to be consumed by fear and anger. I went through so many emotions and I can't recall trying to control the horror that was unfolding before me. I also realized how this must be affecting my little girl. I was on the OR table when I came to this realization. They were on the second attempt at my version. I was allowing my fear of what was now my reality to consume me. Right then and there everything changed.

I was allowed to pick any Pandora station that I wanted and I chose Enya radio. Ever since I was young Enya songs have always been very calming to me. I went into a world that consisted of only me and my baby girl. I spoke to her and I could have sworn that baby spoke back to me. I closed my eyes and began thinking of my little girl who must be as afraid or more than I was. I don't know if I actually heard her or if I could just imagine so vividly what it must be like being in there for her: upside down with a leak in your warm house and your mommy panicking and absolutely in fight or flight mode. I remember almost feeling what she was feeling and I, all of a sudden, felt horrible for causing her to feel that way being so fearful, angry and sorrowful about our current situation. I started talking (in my head) to Zoe (our baby girl), telling her that I was so sorry, that everything was going to be ok and that she didn't have to turn around if she couldn't, we would get her out and be holding her so soon. At that moment I remember going back to the time that I realized that C-sections were indeed a good thing. I knew at that very moment that I loved C-sections. C-sections were going to save my baby's life. They gave me a medication to make my contractions stop, it made me shake uncontrollably. In that moment when I connected with her, I felt a wave of peace flow over me and my shaking stopped.

When the version didn't work, it was ok! I really was ok with it!

Actually I was excited again. I was all smiles and happy tears. We were going to meet our little girl sooner than we thought and we were absolutely, head over heels EXCITED about it!

During my pregnancy, I discussed my fears with my husband and told him about your methods of clearing them. He was on board, but didn't use them. I can remember him being just as heart broken, afraid and upset as I was when we found out that she was breech. He cried to me at one point and repeated over and over again that he was sorry. He felt responsible for protecting both of us and our current circumstances were completely out of his control. When we were in the OR, he was seated behind me holding my hands. I didn't communicate my mental shift but he later told me that he felt it.

The C-section was not scary. I was not afraid anymore. I was happy. Within 15 minutes I held my baby girl. She was perfect!

Every time I tell this story I feel so empowered. I am so thankful that I prepared my mind beforehand. I don't know what would have happened if I hadn't! I found your methods very straight forward. After a while it became effortless. When I noticed that I was worried or frustrated or afraid of anything at all, related or not to my pregnancy, I would confront the issue head on and it was a tremendous help. I have since been digging further into mental health and meditation. I honestly don't know how I made it through this crazy world before without confronting my fears! I feel that I have become a much more confident, strong and happy person because of it!

Thank you for all you do! Grace x

Grace's story is not unique. This is one of many stories I've heard from women who have applied the fearless birthing approach as part of their birth preparation.

Earlier when I asked you to write down your childbirth fears I also asked you to come up with two lists:

1. My *preferred* birth will be like this.....
2. My *least preferred* birth will be like this....

Well, now is the time for us to take what you've written and do something with it. There are two sides to this aspect of the birth preparation:

- Letting go of your *desired* birth outcome
- Making peace with your *least preferred* birth outcome

Letting go

Do you recall the story I shared with you about the lady who shared her traumatic birthing experience, in which she birthed in a hospital and not at home? The birth went well with no problems, but because it didn't take place *where* she wanted it to, she felt traumatised by it. This is a classic case that reminds me of the definition of weeds (plants that are growing in the wrong place). Her birth went well; it just wasn't where she wanted. If she had been able to let go of her need to birth at home, she may well have enjoyed her first few weeks with her new baby instead of experiencing deep grief and loss for an experience she wished she'd had and didn't. If you can *make peace* with not having your ideal birth before you go into labour, you can save yourself a heap of emotional heartache later.

When you're less attached to your birth outcome, if things start to divert off plan you'll be much better placed to go with the flow, which will help to protect the delicate balance of hormones and keep labour moving. Whereas if you respond to things changing with fear or stress, your stress response will slow down labour, which might necessitate medical interventions. The better able you are at going with the flow and staying present, the more likely it is you will have a positive childbirth experience. Remember, situations as they are aren't bad or good, it's our judgement that makes them so.

Letting go of outcomes is one of the easiest ways to live happily and stress-free. When you are no longer hooked on the idea that things or people be a certain way, you open yourself up to enjoy each moment in life and the magic and wonder that may reside in them. If instead of enjoying what you've been given, you're thinking about what you could have had, then you're simply setting yourself up for a fall. Let's nip this one in the bud shall we?

Letting go of certain outcomes is easy - in head trash clearance terms, anyhow - and the more time and effort you spend letting things go in anticipation of unexpected changes, the easier it becomes to do this on the fly. So for the purposes of preparing for your childbirth, you're going to clear the *excess emotional energy* you have around your preferred birthing option. All that "desire" and "want" energy? Yep - that! We're going to clear it out of the way. By lightening your emotional load, you'll be emotionally nimble and better able to respond flexibly to whatever happens on the Big Day.

Making peace

As with letting go of your desired birth, we're going to make peace with your least preferred birthing option by shedding the excess emotional energy you have for the outcome you definitely don't want. So, if you hate the thought of birthing at home, or of having a C-section, once you've done the emotional clearance work, you'll feel less bothered by the thought of a home birth or a C-section. You probably still won't want it, but you'll be more able to see the reasons why it might be a good thing. This is much better than digging your heels in and repeatedly telling yourself in your head that you "Don't want this! Don't want this!" It helps you to get to a place of acceptance more quickly, and in birth, the sooner you're able to do that the better.

Practically speaking

I know I said it was easy to do this clearance work, and I'm not joking. You're basically going to use a slimmed-down version of the *5 Step Head Trash Clearance Method*. Instead of doing mantras for *five* dimensions of head trash, you're only going to do the mantras for *three* of them:

1. The idea of it
2. You experiencing this thing
3. Other people or situations making you experience it

When it comes to using the mantras, you're going to insert the experience you do or don't want into the following mantras:

_____ is a wonderful thing

_____ is a terrible thing

I love _____

I hate _____

I love other people (or events and things) making me
_____ [experience the thing]

I hate other people (or events and things) making me
_____ [experience the thing]

You need to do this for all the things on your list of least preferred birth options and most preferred birth options.

Visualisation

Visualisation is a powerful tool that is known to have a positive effect on outcomes, whether it's a broad life outcome such as achieving your goals, or something specific like birthing your baby. When I talk about visualisation, what I'm NOT talking about are the hypnobirthing visualisations of imagining your cervix as a flower or the contractions as waves. I'm referring to visualisations that will help you to *perform better* during the birthing process.

Visualisation is a well-known and research-backed approach for helping sports people to prepare for and achieve their goals. It is particularly effective at preparing the body, because the mind can't distinguish between an imagined movement and an actual one. So if you "practice" in your mind, it's been shown that the muscles respond better once you do it in reality "because they've already done it". It's a simple premise that has powerful consequences.

So what's stopping us from using this in preparation for birth? Birth is an intensely physical and emotional experience (spiritual too!) and thinking in terms of performance is relevant. You need your body to perform and go the distance, and you need the emotional strength too. Here we can start to draw some similarities with marathon runners. Childbirth is forever being compared to a marathon, so let's take a closer look at how similar they are.

A marathon runner thinks in terms of performance: achieving a certain time, maintaining a pace, etc. To help them succeed, a runner will visualise how calm and relaxed they feel running, how easy they're finding it, how it feels when they pass the finish line. There's no reason why a pregnant woman can't prepare in this way too. You would be hard-pressed to find a runner imagining how painful it's going to be and how it's going to be the most excruciating experience of their life. And you definitely won't find any who are spending their time watching videos of runners having heart attacks or reading statistics on how many people die before they reach the finish line. Why? Because it simply won't help them to succeed.

The magic of visualisation is that it is only limited by your imagination. You can visualise anything you want. The only limit is your mind, which unfortunately can be quite a big limitation, but try not to let it be. It can be too easy for our mind to trick us into limiting what we're imagining by imposing some limiting beliefs on us. So if you're visualising your birth and want to imagine it being pain-free, but your mind jumps in and says, "Oh no! That will never happen! Childbirth is painful. Don't set yourself up for that because you'll only get let down and feel like a failure . . . be realistic!" Well, I say rubbish to that! Put your big-girl pants on for starters.

We know that aiming for something doesn't mean we get it, so don't pile a load of meaning onto your desired outcome. Seriously. Doing this just gives you rope with which to hang yourself later. Don't go there. Visualise your desired outcome, but let go of the outcome too. Don't hang all your life's happiness on it.

The Benefits of Visualisation

Visualisation can do much more than merely help us to achieve our desired outcome.

Stress Relief

Visualisation is a form of relaxation. The simple act of quieting your mind and visualising something can reduce your levels of stress. It's a simple form of meditation that gives your mind a focus and thus prevents the chit-chatter of the mind stressing us out.

Improved Focus

When you take the time to quiet your mind, you're exercising your mind's ability to focus on a single thought. This practice alone is incredibly powerful when it comes to childbirth: the ability to stay totally focussed and not distracted by meddling thoughts and negative emotions. The more you practice the better you become, and you'll notice benefits way beyond birth. Since my children's births, I've noticed how ruthlessly focussed I can be, and I really think that my time spent visualising my childbirths helped me a lot with this.

Boosts Confidence

When we visualise ourselves having and doing the things we want, we begin to feel more confident about ourselves. As we feel more confident, we do more stuff, and this in turn boosts our confidence. So in visualising a positive outcome for your birthing experience, you begin to build confidence in your ability to birth your baby smoothly and safely. This confidence will come with you into childbirth, which will help you to achieve your desired outcome.

Goal Achievement

When we focus our mind on a particular outcome, our subconscious will always be on the lookout for ways to bring us closer to the goal. Maxwell Maltz first drew attention to visualisation as technique for attaining goals in his 1960 book *Psycho-Cybernetics*. He tells us that the word "cybernetics" comes from a Greek term that means "a helmsman who steers his ship to port." "Psycho-cybernetics" is a term he coined, which means "Steering your mind to a productive, useful goal . . . so you can reach the greatest port in the world . . . peace of mind." Nice, don't you think?

In his book he writes, "A human being always acts and feels and performs in accordance with what he imagines to be true about himself and his environment." This is why he encourages using our imagination as the vehicle to bring about personal change. He continues, stating that our brain, nervous system and muscular system are actually "an automatic goal-seeking machine that 'steers' its way to a target or goal by use of feedback data and stored information, automatically correcting the course when necessary." Essentially, what this means is that our mind will seek out a particular goal and self-correct en route. But to do this effectively it needs to be crystal clear on the goal. Just like using your GPS in your car - if you don't input a destination, it just becomes a map. With a destination plugged in, you have a powerful, self-correcting gadget that can take you where you want to go, which is a lot more than a map that simply tells you where you are.

It's worth mentioning at this point what happens if you DON'T set a birth goal for yourself and just go with the flow. Your mind will still pick a thing to aim for, but instead it will pick something from whatever you're focusing on. Let's imagine you decide that your birth prep strategy is going to consist mainly of watching *One Born Every Minute* and you end up watching loads of scary births. Your mind will interpret that as your goal. After all, you're spending so much time focusing on it, why wouldn't it be? When you're about to go on holiday, do you spend the weeks beforehand watching documentaries on planes crashing and people arriving on their holiday to half built hotels? Probably not.

Prepares the Body

The act of practicing and rehearsing in your mind is a brilliant way for your body to practice doing something. The mind can't tell between something that is imagined or real, so by taking the time to practice imagining doing something physical, you're enabling your body to practice doing the thing you want to achieve. Athletes and musicians use this technique all the time. A scientific study[30] was conducted on athletes looking to improve their free throws in basketball; they were divided into three groups:

- Group 1: Physically took practice free throw shots during the day
- Group 2: Only visualised making shots every day
- Group 3: Physically took practice free throw shots during the day, and before going to bed they visualised making perfect shots

Here's what happened:

- Group 1 (only took shots): Improved free throw shooting by 7%
- Group 2 (only visualised making shots): Improved free throw shooting by 10%
- Group 3 (took shots and visualised making shots): Improved free throw shooting by 32%

The results speak for themselves.

To get the best results

The best results come when you aren't trying too hard or expecting too much. As I hinted at earlier, it's a bit of a paradox: you have to let go of what you want in order to improve your chances of getting it. Ideally, you should approach your visualisation exercises as pleasant and relaxing, and let go of wondering whether they will "work" or not.

To give your visualisations extra oomph, involve as many of your senses as possible. This means using sight, sound, smell, and feeling to really create an impactful visualisation. Importantly, you need to imagine you doing the thing as if you are actually doing it, not watching yourself doing it. This is sometimes described as *associated* (feeling like you're doing it), as opposed to *dissociated* (say, watching yourself on TV doing it). So imagine what you will see through your eyes, what smells and sounds you might notice, what sensations you will notice in your body, and how you will be feeling emotionally.

Visualising your birth

As we bring all this together, think about how this might work when it comes to birth. You might want to consider:

- HOW your birthing experience will go: take time to imagine your childbirth and how you'd like it to unfold. *Smoothly? Safely? Fast or slow? Long or short? Effortless? Painless?*
- How you will FEEL: *Confident? Happy? Calm? Relaxed? Full of joy? Excited? Strong? Empowered? Euphoric?*
- How your baby will feel: *Trusting in you? Confident in themselves?*

You might want to visualise some details like having a home birth or a water birth, but be careful with this, because if you don't get your home or water birth, you might get in an emotional tangle. This is where it's important to let go of our desired outcomes (more on this in a bit). This is an ideal exercise for your partner to undertake too, so be sure to share your visualisations with your partner.

In the lead-up to my second childbirth I used visualisations a lot. In the final five weeks or so, I must have visualised every day. I decided with my second birth that I wanted it to be smooth and quick. I'd read that second births tend to be about half as long as first births, so I aimed for a three-hour birth (my first was six hours).

In my visualisations, I would bring clear visuals into my mind and narrate to myself. This was partly to give words to things, but also a way of communicating with my baby and letting her know how I'd like things to go. This was so that we were both on the same page! The main things I focussed my visualisations on were the ideas of my birth being smooth, quick, safe, and painless. I envisioned me birthing effortlessly and just getting on with it in a focussed manner, like I had an important job that needed to be done. Which I did! In my visualisations I noticed how calm and relaxed I felt and how I was enjoying birthing my baby.

We were planning a home birth and we had bought a birthing pool for me to use during labour, but I never visualised me being in the pool. In fact I didn't notice a location or a position in my visualisations. Instead I focussed my visualisation on how I was feeling emotionally, and how my body was feeling. In hindsight, this was a good thing as the birth was so quick that the pool wasn't ready in time!

Incredibly, the birth I had was the birth I visualised. When the midwife announced the time of the earthside arrival of my daughter, it was two hours and fifty-eight minutes after labour had begun. My daughter appeared out of nowhere and caught us all by surprise. I suddenly stood up and the midwife asked if I wanted to push. I said yes and out she came. I still had my pyjamas on and we were scrambling to pull them down to let her out. I love to think my little one suddenly noticed the time and realised that she was due out and just ejected herself to stay on schedule with our agreed plan.

Waiting for Baby

As you approach the arrival of your baby, the one thing that will help you is to remain calm and free of stress. However, this is much easier said than done. It's a strange limbo time wherein you're caught between two phases of your life. If your baby arrives early, you miss out on a lot of this, but if you sail past your due date, remaining calm is not always easy, as I've already talked about.

I decided to create a podcast episode to help women who are due any day. I originally did it because I was inspired by one of my podcast listeners, Alia. When I decided to touch base with Alia around her due date, she replied to let me know that I was emailing her ON HER DUE DATE! Her little mister still hadn't made an appearance, but she was feeling great and looking forward to the birth. When I replied to her, I immediately thought of lots of things I wanted to say, but it was late and I was supposed to be turning the light out and going to sleep, so I kept it short. But in the morning, I thought that I'd still like to share some words with her and then it hit me: why not turn it into a podcast? You can listen to it here.

Here are some of key things that really helped me remain calm in the stressful lead-up to my second birth:

Be Patient

I know this bit can be really hard. We can't help it; we have a due date in our heads and for months we focus on it, waiting for that day to arrive. It symbolises such a momentous event - the actual birth, meeting our little one, becoming a mother (again, maybe), saying goodbye to our old life, welcoming the new. This is BIG! And yet we don't know exactly when it's going to unfold. It feels like it's all being done *to you* and you have no choice. Towards the end, you can feel pretty fed up with the whole pregnancy thing and you just want it to end. The trick here is be mindful and stay in the present. Sounds easier than it is, I know! But if you focus on anything other than the here and now, it simply makes it harder. Enjoy this limbo time.

Create a Bubble of Positive Calmness for Yourself

Try to start disconnecting from the real world, especially social media, and start going *within*. This calmness before the storm won't last long, so claim it while you can. This is when we reap the benefits of telling people a due *month*, or adding a couple of weeks to the due date that you share with people so you won't be getting all those texts and Facebook messages asking for updates.

Connect and Talk to Your Baby

Some people find this hard, but it's actually very simple. Find a quiet spot for you to be undisturbed. Maybe sitting under a tree at the park, on a lounger in the garden, or at home on a load of cushions. Once you're comfy, start to feel your baby through your belly. Maybe apply a bit of pressure to your bump to let them know you'd like to chat, and then just start talking! You can do this in your head if you want; it doesn't really matter. What matters is the intention and the feeling that lies behind what you're saying. Your baby is part of you and shares your body. Of course your baby can tell what's going on in your mind!

Here are some of the things that I was saying to my little one while I was waiting for her to make an appearance:

How are you?

I'm really looking forward to meeting you!

Are you ready to come out?

I'd just like to share with you how I'd like our birth
to go . . .

You, me, and my body know exactly how to do this, so it
should all be fine.

I totally trust you and my body to be able to bring you
out safely and smoothly.

I know that the best thing for me to do is step aside and
let you two run the show . . . but I'll be there if you
need me to . . . you know that, right?

It's going to be painless for both of us . . . there's no need
to worry. I'm saying that for my benefit too, by
the way!

We're going to enjoy it . . . it's exciting! I bet you're
excited . . . I am!

Daddy CANNOT WAIT to meet you! He's going to be
the first person that you touch . . . how's that for a
welcome!

We're going to be able to look back on your arrival with
joy and happiness

Now, I've heard that second births are half as long as first
births, so this means that you might show up in three
hours. I'm totally cool with that. In fact, a short birth
would be nice. So how about we wrap this whole
thing up in three hours? Yep? I'm up for that if you
are. There's no point in dragging this thing out. You
know what you're doing and my body knows what
it's doing. As long as I get out the way, this shouldn't
be a problem. Yep? Cool.

MOVE!

Keep moving! It doesn't have to be massively exhausting and energetic. Even if you're sitting around on your Swiss ball gyrating and having a bounce to some music. I remember listening to two rounds of my favourite dance music radio show, while in a hypnotic trance on the day before Baby arrived. I was bouncing, swaying, and getting up every now and then for a dance. Looking back, it was six hours that just flew by. I had no idea I was doing it for that long!

Maybe go for walks, or do some yoga . . . just something to connect to your body. You're going to be working as a team soon, so create that connection as best you can.

And finally, just remember:

You've got this!

Remember to trust that your body KNOWS what to do.

Your body is MADE for doing this. It will not let you down . . . as long as you trust in the process and surrender to it.

Good luck!

Resources that Accompany this Book

As I've mentioned throughout this book, I have created some resources to help you on your fearless birthing journey. These include:

- Your FREE fear-clearance meditation mp3
- PDF downloads to accompany the exercises in the book

To access the resources area sign up here:
fearless-birthing.com/book-resources

Can I Support You?

If you would like me to support you on your journey to motherhood, then book a free chat today.

To book some time for us to speak please visit http://alexialeachman.com/book-chat

Send me an email!

If you would like to email me then feel free to send an email to

alexia@fearfreechidbirth.com

I love receiving listener and reader emails!

References

1. CL Pasero and R Britt (August 1998) "Managing Pain During Labor" published in the American Journal of Nursing 98:10–11
2. Van de Carr & Lehrer, 1986
3. Van de Carr, Van de Carr & Lehrer, 1988
4. Manrique et al., 1993
5. Carlson & Labarba, 1979; Connally & Cullen, 1983; Ferreira, 1965; Montagu, 1962; Stott, 1957
6. Zuckerman, Bauchner, Parker, & Cabrai, 1990
7. Feldman, 1981
8. Ward, 1991
9. National Center for Child Health and Development, Allergy Division in Tokyo. Geneva, Switzerland, June 17, 2012
10. NICE Costing Report November 2011. www.nice.org.uk/guidance/cg132/resources/costing-report-184766797
11. Calculating Due Dates and the Impact of Mistaken Estimates of Gestational Age www.transitiontoparenthood.com//ttp/birthed/duedatespaper.htm

12. Morken, Melve and Skjaerven (2011)
13. Mendelson 2009
14. Stanford Medicine Magazine. Pain's Stronghold - It's All in Your Head, Fall 2005.
http://sm.stanford.edu/archive/stanmed/2005fall/pain.html
15. Dread and the Disvalue of Future Pain (November 21, 2013)
http://journals.plos.org/ploscompbiol/article?id=10.1371/journal.pcbi.1003335
16. New Scientist. Waiting for pain can cause more dread than pain itself (November 2013)
https://www.newscientist.com/article/dn24642-waiting-for-pain-can-cause-more-dread-than-pain-itself/
17. (Robertson, 1999).
18. National Vital Statistics Report. Volume 63, Number 6.
https://www.cdc.gov/nchs/data/nvsr/nvsr63/nvsr63_06.pdf
19. World Health Organization. World Health Report (2010) Background Paper, 30.
http://who.int/healthsystems/topics/financing/healthreport/30C-sectioncosts.pdf
20. US National Library of Medicine National Institute for Health. Manuscript PMC2475575. Neonatal Morbidity and Mortality After Elective Cesarean Delivery
https://www.ncbi.nlm.nih.gov/pmc/articles/PMC2475575/
21. US National Library of Medicine National Institute for Health. Manuscript PMC2730905. Safe, Healthy Birth: What Every Pregnant Woman Needs to Know.
http://www.ncbi.nlm.nih.gov/pmc/articles/PMC2730905/
22. Sakala & Corry, 2008
23. Storton, 2007
24. Birth, June 1986, Letters, 124–125
25. Hill, Piatt & Manning, 1979; Manning, Piatt & Lemay 1977; Neldam & Pedersen, 1980; Ron & Polishuk, 1976

26. Birnholz, Stephens & Faria, 1978
27. Baker, 1978
28. James Clear. How Long Does it Actually Take to Form a New Habit (Backed by Science)
    http://jamesclear.com/new-habit
29. European Journal of Social Psychology. How habits are formed: Modelling habit formation in the real world (July 2009).
    http://onlinelibrary.wiley.com/doi/10.1002/ejsp.674/abstract
30. Breakthrough Basketball. Mental Rehearsal and Visualiszation. The secret to improving your game without touching a basketball.
    https://www.breakthroughbasketball.com/mental/visualization.html

Acknowledgments

Huge gratitude to Chris Milbank, the rebellious genius and inspiration who founded Reflective Repatterning, and who encouraged me to take it forth into the world and make it my own. Thank you for your guidance, inspiration, wisdom and healing.

This book is the result of many small moments that I could have easily ignored or let pass without thinking. But for whatever reason, I didn't. Together they've brought me here and have had a huge impact on me and the direction of my life and work.

Thank you Pam Lidford. I'll always remember our lunch in London when you told me about the course that would change my life.

Thank you to Julie Watkins, for innocently diverting me on to the right track as you tried to make me feel better about being pregnant and fearful.

My aunt and beloved spiritual mentor, Nicole Goldman, who planted the seed that this is the book I needed to write (and not the other one I was so sure of). Merci Nicole, pour tout!

Thank you to Lisa Young for asking me how I did it. Your email forced me to really think about what I did and how I did it. You being pregnant gave me the pressure I needed to get cracking.

Once, the first draft was complete, I was blessed with the support and patience of some wonderful friends who gave way more than they needed to, including but by no way limited to:

Steff Spencer. Thanks for your endless support and kicks up the ass. And for doing what all good friends should do: highlighting to me the head trash I need to work on!

Shaun Hopkins. Thank you for reading and re-reading a book which wasn't exactly something you'd normally read. Thank you for your time, your honesty, your guidance and your support.

Mark Shaw. Thank you for selflessly giving your time in reading early versions of my book and letting me know that my writing was not too shabby. Coming from you, that meant a lot. I'm so sorry you can't be here to read the final manuscript. Thank you for our day with Prince Harry. It's not one I'll ever forget!

Catherine Holland. Your support and cheerleading has helped me more than you know. This is just the beginning!

Andy Briscoe, who in my mind is the best designer you could ever wish for. Thank you SO much for offering to step in when I needed it. It means more to me than you could ever know. And this cover, is quite simply perfect!

I want to give a huge thank you to my podcast listeners and to the members of my Facebook group. Your emails, posts and questions have helped me to refine my first draft into the book I've finally birthed. I've learned so much from you and I'm so grateful for your support and cheerleading.

And finally, I want to thank and appreciate those who have played much bigger roles in my life. *Thank* feels like such a small word, but for me it's a big, fabulous word filled with love and gratitude;

Eternal gratitude to my mother. Losing you was the wake up call I needed to be me and get on track. It hasn't been an easy ride, but I think I'm getting there. I miss you more than you can imagine. You inspire me every day.

Bruce, my rock. Thank you for being you and being there, for your patience and trusting that I could do this.

Lila & Sofia. Thank you for choosing me to be your mother and for the joy and laughter you bring me each day.

Meet the Fearless Birthing Family

Fearless Birthing Academy

This is the online programme that supports the *Fearless Birthing* book. It brings all of the chapters alive through videos, audios, workbooks and other downloads to help you prepare for your positive birth experience. If you're committed to your Fearless Birthing journey and need extra help to make it happen, this online program is for you.

Find out more at

fearless-birthing.com/academy

Fearless Mama Ship

This is the ultimate online resource to help you to prepare for the transition to motherhood. It includes a Fearless Birth Prep program that walks you through Alexia's essential steps of birth prep as well as an extensive library of information and inspiration to support you through your four trimesters. There are interviews with midwives and birth experts, bonus podcast episodes, downloadable birth plans and video series.

Find out more at

fearless-birthing.com/fearless-mama-ship

Tokophobia Support Program

This is Alexia's specialist program for women with tokophobia that is based on her Fearless Birthing Academy program. It's an online program that is combined with calls with Alexia to offer additional levels of support.

www.fearfreechildbirth.com/tokophobia-support-program/

Professional Training

If you're interested in learning the Head Trash Clearance Method to use with your clients, Alexia offers the following training courses:

Fearless Birthing Professional Training

Learn the Fearless Birthing method and join the tribe of Fearless Birthing Professionals. This training is for doulas, midwives, pregnancy and birth therapists, and other professionals who serve and support growing families.

Visit fearless-birthing.com/training for more information

Head Trash Clearance Method Training

If you're a therapist, counsellor or coach and would like to learn the Head Trash Clearance Method so that you can use it with your clients visit

headtrash.co.uk/practitioner-training/

About the Author

Alexia is a therapeutic coach and host of the award-nominated and chart-topping *Fear Free Childbirth* podcast. What began as a maternity leave side project is now an essential destination for women with a fear of birth with thousands of expectant mamas now using Alexia's site to lose The Fear and prepare for birth.

It all started when Alexia experienced her first miscarriage and felt relief; she knew something was amiss. She had tokophobia, the extreme fear of pregnancy and birth, which is pretty terrifying. Alexia used her superpowers to overcome it and have two amazing births, and she now helps other women do the same with her private sessions, her online programmes and products, and of course her podcast.

Alexia lives in the middle of England with her partner and their two daughters.

www.alexialeachman.com

Also by Alexia Leachman

Clear Your Head Trash

How to Create Clarity, Peace & Confidence in Your Life & Work

Clear Your Head Trash is your essential road map to confront and conquer the fears, stresses and anxieties that prevent you from thinking clearly, doing your best and living with confidence. Through Leachman's unique Head Trash Clearance Method, you'll discover how to reclaim your headspace so that you can get on with enjoying your life and work.

In Clear Your Head Trash, you'll discover

- The Head Trash Clearance Method, that you can use to rid your fears, anxieties and stresses
- How stop being emotionally triggered by day-to-day life situations
- Where the destructive patterns and habits in your life come from, and how to tackle them
- How to streamline your thoughts and feelings so that you can think more clearly and feel calmer
- How to address the unpleasant emotions in your life and move on from them more easily

Clear Your Head Trash is a must-read for anyone who is serious about their personal development. The clearance method shared in this book has been changing lives for years… and now it's your turn.

Publisher: Mankai Media; 1st ed. 2018

Ebook: 978-1-9998915-2-7

Paperback: 978-1-9998915-3-4

Alexia has contributed to the following book;

Childbirth, Midwifery & the Media

This edited collection - one of a kind in its field - addresses the theoretical and practical implications facing representations of midwifery and media. Bringing together international scholars and practitioners, this succinct volume offers a cross-disciplinary discussion regarding the role of media in childbirth, midwifery and pregnancy representation. One chapter critiques the provision and dissemination of health information and promotional materials in a suburban antenatal clinic, while others are devoted to specific forms of media – television, the press, social media – looking at how each contribute to women's perceptions and anxieties with regard to childbirth.

Publisher: Palgrave Macmillan; 1st ed. 2017 edition (5 Nov. 2017)

ISBN-10: 3319635123

ISBN-13: 978-3319635125

CPSIA information can be obtained
at www.ICGtesting.com
Printed in the USA
BVHW041304100119
537533BV00013B/89/P